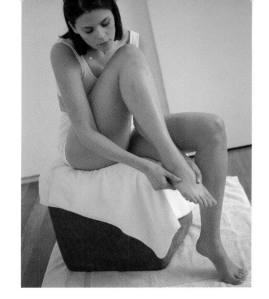

AYURVEDA

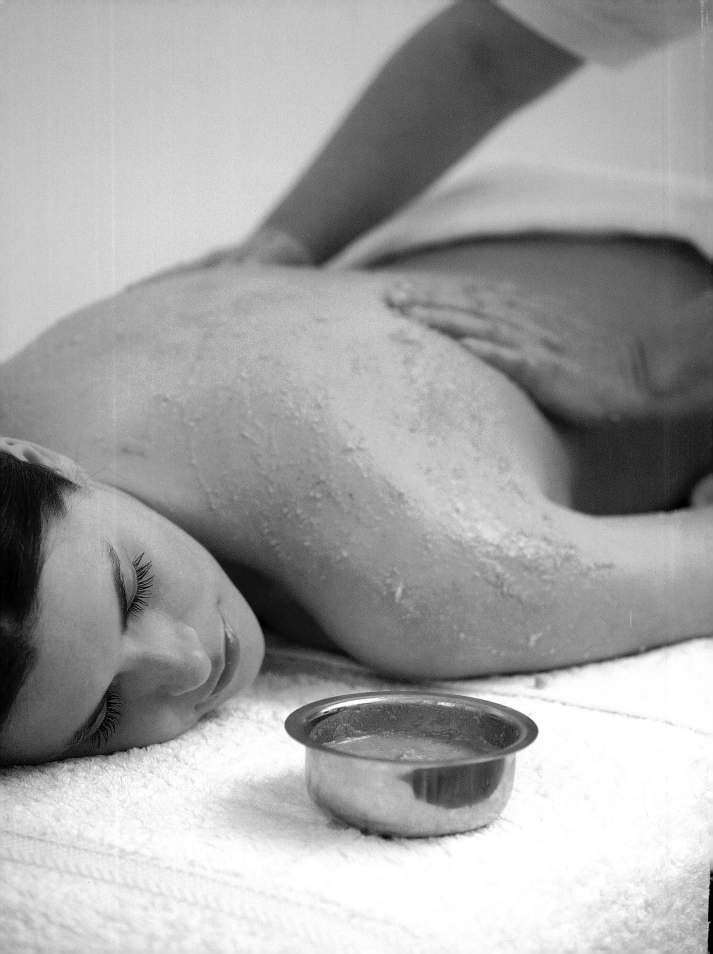

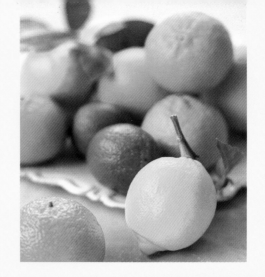

AYURVEDA

ANNA SELBY
CONSULTANT IAN HAYWARD

DISCOVER THE
SECRETS OF
AYURVEDA TO
BALANCE YOUR
MIND, BODY
AND SOUL

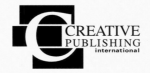

CREATIVE
PUBLISHING
international

For Christian, as ever.

Published in the USA and Canada in 2001 by
Creative Publishing international, Inc.

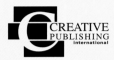

Creative Publishing international, Inc.
5900 Green Oak Drive
Minnetonka, Minnesota 55343

First published in Great Britain in 2001 by
Collins & Brown Limited
London House
Great Eastern Wharf
Parkgate Road
London SW11 4NQ

9 8 7 6 5 4 3 2 1

ISBN 1-58923-017-5

Commissioned by Grace Cheetham
Art directed by Anne-Marie Bulat
Project managed by Clare Churly
Edited by Beth Simms
Designed by Sue Miller
Photography by Winfried Heinze and Nicki Dowey

Reproduction by Global Colour, Malaysia
Printed and bound in Singapore by Craft Print International Ltd

This book was typeset using Blur, Rockwell and Gill Sans.

Safety note
The information in this book is not intended as a
substitute for medical advice. Any person suffering from
conditions requiring medical attention, or who has
symptoms that concern them, should consult a qualified
medical practitioner.

Contents

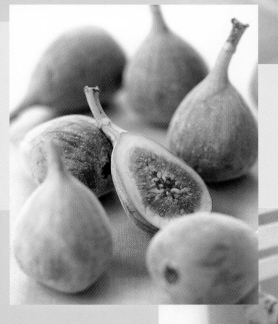

Introduction

Ayurveda is one of the most ancient systems of healthcare we know of. It was first established at least 5,000 years ago and has been in continual use ever since. It is now recognized as the basis of all the Eastern forms of medicine and perhaps, too, the very roots of Western medicine. It is still the most widely used healthcare system in India and is recognized by the World Health Organization as one of the principal healing disciplines.

Ayurveda means, literally, science of life: "ayu" being the Sanskrit word for "life" and "veda" for "knowledge." As its name suggests, ayurveda is a body of knowledge—of wisdom—that covers all aspects of our lives and it is holistic in the true sense of the word. Unlike allopathic—Western—medicine, which has traditionally addressed itself to the relief of symptoms, ayurveda not only aims to eradicate the underlying causes of disease, it begins from an altogether deeper level, creating a balance within body and soul that acts as an effective defense against illness.

Prevention rather than cure

In ayurveda, the prevention of disease is even more important than its cure. In the West, we are used to a mechanistic attitude to the body, regarding it as something to be repaired when it breaks down, as we would a piece of machinery. We are used to taking medicine or undergoing surgery to counter a very specific illness or symptom. As a result, some of ayurveda's preventive methods may seem strange at first. As complementary and holistic therapies have become increasingly popular, most of us are more aware that a beneficial diet and exercise are vital for maintaining good health. In addition to these disciplines ayurveda includes those that might initially seem quite unconnected to your health: for example, meditation, the way you pace your day, breathing techniques and establishing a different relationship with nature.

According to ayurveda, however, just about everything is connected to your state of health. Not only does it see you in a holistic light—there are no barriers between body, mind and spirit in ayurveda—it sees you as a part of the environment, nature and the universe beyond. For you to be healthy and content, you must be in harmony not just within yourself but with the world around you.

Harmony and balance: these are the starting points of ayurveda and the place to which it always returns. The principle is easy enough to grasp—after all, people who are at ease with themselves and those around them are generally happier and less prone to stress than those who are at odds with the world. Ayurveda turns this sense of harmony into a goal that you can move toward, step by step, as you develop an understanding and experience of how the mind and body work and of some basic laws of nature. As you begin to look at life and nature through ayurvedic eyes, you see it in quite a different way. And, though the underlying precepts may seem simple and straightforward, they can revolutionize your health and sense of well-being to a profound degree.

Ayurveda in the West

Given the potency of ayurveda, then, it may seem strange that it has so far had little impact in the West. There are a number of reasons for this. Under British rule, Western medical practices were introduced in India and many Indians began to regard ayurveda as a second-class form of health-care at best—and, at worst, little more than super-stition. Given the low esteem in which it was held by Indians, there was little chance of it becoming more highly regarded away from the land of its birth.

In recent years, however, certain ayurvedic practitioners and teachers (notably the Maharishi, Deepak Chopra, Vasant Lad and David Frawley) have gone back to the original teachings of the rishis (the enlightened sages of the ancient vedic texts). At last, this highly sophisticated and effective system of healthcare has emerged from the shad-ows of folklore to enjoy a timely revival. However, in the West it has still not caught on in quite the way that might have been expected. The reason for this is that it is still regarded as being part of a very Indian philosophy and way of life. Westerners imagine that ayurveda necessitates changing to an Indian diet, undergoing dire, purgative treatments, adopting at least the lotus position, if not an entire religion and culture. Not surprisingly, this is more of a change than most of us are keen to make.

European ayurveda

None of these radical changes is needed, however, because ayurveda is universal. And this is where European ayurveda (EAV)—the health spas and this book—comes in, interpreting this vast body of knowledge for the West. Without diluting the core,

underlying principles, EAV aims to make the ben-efits of ayurveda available and accessible to Westerners by adapting its precepts to the Western way of life. The natural laws that operate in the West are subtly different than those in India—its cli-mate, culture and social conditions. For instance, in a system of healthcare in which the rhythms of the seasons play an integral part, we need to look at the climate that exists in the place where we live. Ayurveda traditionally includes the monsoon—something that few of us in the West experience.

Similarly, over many generations, our digestive systems have evolved to cope with different kinds of food. The Indian diet includes much more oil and ghee than most Westerners could comfortably cope with and it would be unrealistic—and not par-ticularly profitable in health terms—for us simply to adopt wholesale the diet of the subcontinent. Instead, EAV recommends food from your own environment and culture because you are a part of it, just as it is a part of you.

There is no need, either, to tie our limbs in knots in order to be able to meditate or practice yoga, and nor do we have to change our belief system in order to make ayurveda work for us. Ayurveda is, above all, a natural philosophy. In our frantically busy and high-tech world, it puts us back in touch with both our own physiology and the rhythms of the world around us.

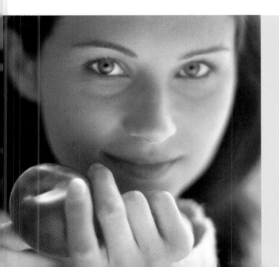

There are no barriers between body, mind and spirit in ayurveda – it sees you as a part of the environment, nature and the universe beyond.

How to use this book

This book explains ayurveda and the concepts of an ayurvedic health spa, and shows you how you can incorporate these into your life. It is not a book to put away and display on the shelf – it is one you can use every day.

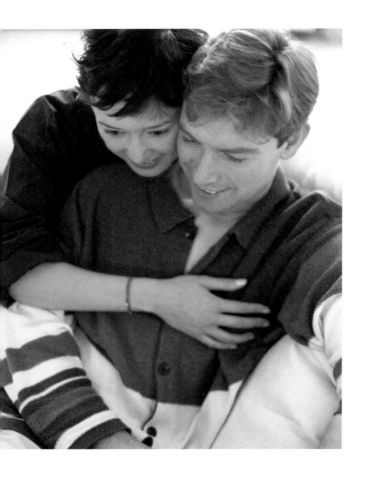

Ayurveda does not attempt to treat serious conditions—in such cases you should always consult a qualified medical practitioner. However, it can make a profound difference to your health and well-being, alleviating long-standing chronic conditions, improving your state of mind, reducing stress, and enhancing your immune function and your energy levels.

So how can ayurveda work for you? In many ways, that depends on what you need. This is not an evasion. Unlike most health disciplines, ayurveda does not stipulate one rule for all. On the contrary, it sees us all as individuals. Depending upon your physiological type—your doshic makeup—ayurveda will recommend a diet, an exercise routine and a pattern to your day that are tailored for you as an individual. So you need to begin by understanding the doshas and identifying your own mind and body type using the questionnaire and analysis on pages 32–9. Answer all the questions as honestly as you can, being careful to differentiate between your normal state of body and mind and any current conditions. Use the answers to assess your prakriti (combination of doshas) and any imbalance you may have, and then read on to the parts of the book that particularly apply to you.

When you start putting the ideas of this book into practice and make even small changes, you will begin to see immediate benefits; the more changes that you make, the more you will start to find your own inner balance. You will also begin to recognize when you don't have that sense of balance—when you feel out of sorts, physically, mentally or emotionally. Having gained this deeper insight into the way you function, you will be able, too, to work out the cause of the problem, be it eating unsuitable foods, lack of sleep or an unsettling factor in your environment or relationships.

This process whereby you begin to be able to put yourself back in balance is known as self-referral and it is the key to this book. It puts you in control of yourself and your health, and eventually leads you to the happy state in which you know instinctively how to maintain an inner harmony of body and soul, known in EAV as spontaneous right action.

1 In Part One, the basics of European ayurveda are explained and you will learn how to identify your own prakriti.

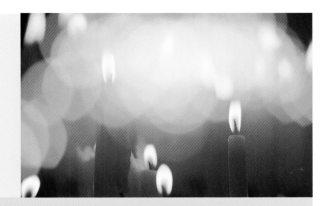

2 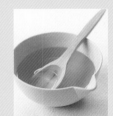 The second part of the book, "Your home spa," reveals ayurvedic spa principles for your daily life. "The food spa" finds the best diet for your health, "The body spa" introduces you to ayurvedic exercise and "The mind spa" shows you how you can learn to relax and unleash the power and creativity of your own mind to help you get the most out of life on every level. "The treatment spa" gives an introduction to the luxurious treatments of European ayurveda, including your own deeply beneficial self-massage.

3 The third part of the book looks at ayurveda in a wider context. It shows you how to understand your doshic makeup and make the most of it at work, at play and in your own home environment, so that all of your surroundings and activities support it. In effect, it is an all-of-your-life spa!

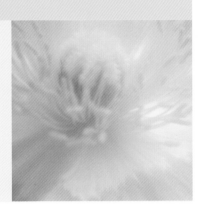

how the color coding works

Throughout the book you will see that each of the doshas is identified by a different color – vata is green, pitta is blue and kapha is red. You can use this color-coding to turn instantly to the information that is relevant to your own doshic makeup.

vata

pitta

kapha

PART ONE

Perfect balance

Your body has its own inner intelligence, the sole purpose of which is to keep you healthy. Every night while you sleep, it processes toxins, removes dead and damaged cells and replaces them with new healthy ones. However, when you overload yourself with too much stress and too little sleep, junk food, alcohol and drugs, your body has to deal with these toxins before it can begin to heal and rejuvenate. Over time, your body's ability to repair itself is weakened and, according to ayurveda, this is the point at which you become vulnerable to illness and unhappiness. However, the opposite effect can be achieved too. It is on this level that ayurveda has a unique wisdom, putting the mind and body back into balance and preventing the onset of symptoms and eventual disease by stimulating your own inner defenses.

Chapter one
Nature's building blocks

Health is more than a mere absence of disease. If you enjoy good health to its fullest, you not only lack any specific ailment, you have inner resources of energy and immunity and you feel content mentally and emotionally. Unfortunately, although we do sometimes experience this glowing state of health, few of us can maintain it permanently, living as we do in a state of constant change.

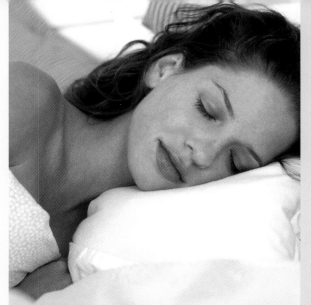

Vata people

Elements:
air and ether

Nature:
wind and ocean

Colors:
ocher and yellow

Sounds:
silence, chanting or
quiet, calming music

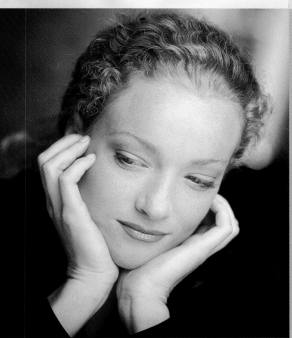

Pitta people

Elements:
fire and water

Nature:
fire and the heat of
the sun

Colors:
blue and violet

Sounds:
soft, calm music,
the sound of the
sea, waterfalls and
running water

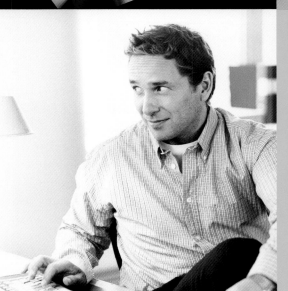

Kapha people

Elements:
earth and water

Nature:
rocks, mountains
and the earth

Colors:
red and orange

Sounds:
loud, fast music

Good health

Your state of health can, in fact, be affected by many different factors. Your general physical condition and your ability to resist disease depend on your diet and lifestyle, as well as on your state of mind. External factors—the weather, pollution, your living and working environments—will affect you too.

On a daily basis, the pattern of your life can change: you stay up late and get only a few hours' sleep, you spend an evening in a smoky atmosphere, you take a flight and change time zones. All of these seemingly unimportant events can have a subtle effect on your physiology.

From an ayurvedic point of view, disease is not simply the opposite of health, the two being distinct, discrete states. Instead, ayurveda has a sliding scale with many gradations, in which minor imbalances need to be addressed to prevent them from turning into symptoms that, in turn, can become diseases. This is a very different approach to health and illness than the allopathic (Western) method.

Traditional Western medicine seeks to identify the offending pathogen and administer the appropriate drug to disarm or eradicate it. This is the magic-bullet approach that most of us in the developed world take for granted. In fact, this form of treatment is now so universal that many people feel their condition has not been taken seriously if they leave their doctor's office without a prescription. It is an approach that essentially sees people very much as machines—and if one part of the machine fails, it can be fixed or even replaced.

By contrast, ayurveda regards good health as the result of a harmonious inner balance. Nature itself—our own body—is the healer and ayurveda aims to strengthen that inner balance so that healing takes place naturally and effectively. There are, of course, many ayurvedic remedies—and even surgery—available from qualified ayurvedic physicians if you are suffering from a serious condition.

However, ideally, ayurveda prevents both symptoms and diseases from taking hold by redressing imbalances at the earliest possible stage. This entails forgoing the firing of magic bullets and instead embracing the bigger picture—therefore taking more responsibility for your own health than most of us are used to doing.

Boosting immunity

A room full of people can be exposed to a virus for the same amount of time and in the same conditions but only some of them will succumb to it. Why? If the external conditions are the same for them all, it can only be that the internal conditions are what makes the difference.

Our ability to resist both external infection and internal degenerative disease depends on the strength of our immune system, and in the sophisticated developed world our immune systems are under constant attack. We live life at a hectic pace, work for long hours in demanding jobs, run homes, bring up children and try to find time for a social life. We become tired and run-down, never feeling on top of things, and, because time is the one thing most of us don't have enough of, we cut corners. We eat convenience, or junk, food, suffer from lack of sleep, feel guilty about never making it to the gym, and drink too much or smoke as a quick-fix way to wind down. Of course, we all know this is no way to live, but we still carry on doing it—perhaps because we don't realize quite how much damage we are doing to ourselves.

Our bodies are extremely complex organisms in a state of constant growth and renewal on a cellular level. They get rid of old, damaged and dead cells and replace them with new ones on a daily basis. The metabolism has its own system of priorities. If we fall ill, our body concentrates its energies on repelling invading infections and on the healing process.

When we subject ourselves to endless stress and toxins, these are treated as a similarly urgent priority and our bodies work on rendering them harmless. However, while our bodies are busy defusing these potential triggers, they have less energy for the everyday processes of cleansing, healing and renewal. Over time, the body can't keep up the pace, the strain shows on the overworked organs and systems and the body's performance—its ability to protect itself from disease—slows down.

Clearly, this process takes time and it may be years before you become aware of a problem. However, when you do become aware of a problem, your immune system will already have been undermined and you will have come, step by step, a long way from that picture of glowing good health with which we began. At this point, there may be no alternative to the magic bullet.

If you take the ayurvedic path, however, your focus will be on establishing a protective inner balance, not by relying on magic bullets but by making small changes gradually in your diet, your exercise routine, your lifestyle and your attitudes. Because we are all different and we all change constantly through the seasons and as we grow older, these changes differ too, from person to person. It is how we adapt to this constant change that is important.

Ayurveda regards **good health** as the result of a harmonious inner balance. Nature itself—our **own body**—is the healer and ayurveda aims to strengthen that **inner balance** so that healing takes place **naturally** and effectively.

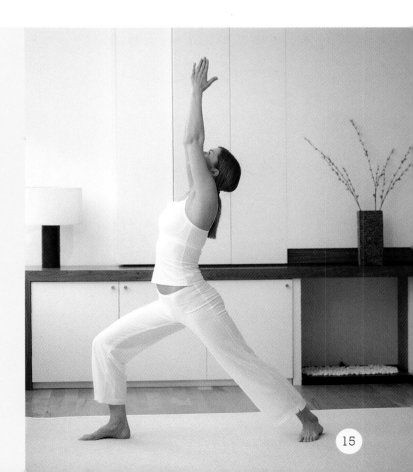

The three doshas

In ayurveda, the world is divided into doshas—vata, pitta and kapha. There is no exact translation in English, but doshas can be regarded as vital energies or principles that underlie everything we are, everything we think or do, and everything around us.

Each of us has a unique doshic makeup (prakriti) in which one or more of the three is dominant within us. Nevertheless, we all contain all three doshas in varying amounts. We are born with our particular doshic constitution, depending on our parents' prakritis at the time of conception and on our mothers' experiences during pregnancy. From the moment we are born, however, our prakritis are affected by everything that goes on around us and everything we ourselves do. When our doshas are upset and out of balance, our health and sense of well-being suffer. This does not, incidentally, mean that all three doshas are evenly balanced. It means that they are balanced according to our individual doshic constitution—that we are essentially in a state of inner harmony which is unique to each and every one of us. However, the doshas pertain to much more than human beings; they are underlying principles that apply to the world around us, as the following pages reveal.

As you will see in this chapter, the doshas are the fundamental life energies, extending not only to every part of our minds and bodies, but to the world around us too. It would be wrong, though, to see them as static. The doshas are, like life itself, always in transition.

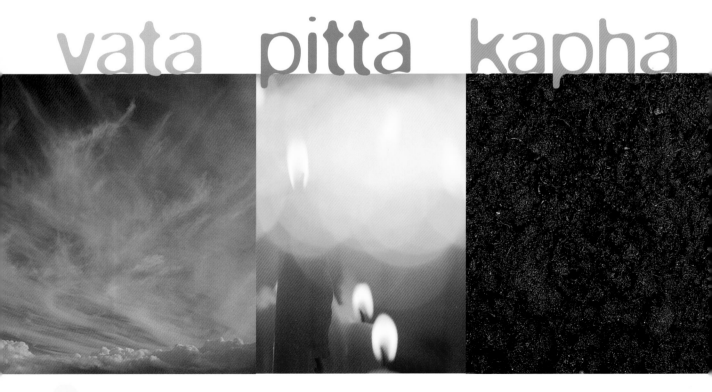

vata   pitta   kapha

Balancing the doshas

At different times of day and year and at different stages in our lives, one of the doshas predominates before it yields to another. Certain kinds of foods, weather conditions and activities also have a particular doshic quality and will serve to increase, or aggravate, one dosha, while decreasing, or pacifying, another.

Just as the world around us is constantly changing, so we too are always in transition. This is a perfectly natural rhythm and it is of concern only when one dosha is sufficiently aggravated to become imbalanced.

When a particular dosha is increased, it can be pacified by food, actions or environments that have the opposite qualities to its own. For instance, vata's qualities include coldness and movement. If you have a vata imbalance and the day has vata qualities —it is cold and windy, say—you can pacify vata by wrapping up in warm clothes, taking particular care of your head and ears, keeping indoors as much as possible, and having warm, nourishing food and drinks. If, on the other hand, you spend hours out in this kind of weather in skimpy clothes, and drink gassy, iced drinks at the same time, vata will soar.

Similarly, one of pitta's main qualities is heat. If you have a pitta imbalance, spending most of your time in overheated conditions—whether sunbathing or slaving over a hot stove—will aggravate your pitta, as will hot, spicy foods. On the other hand, going for a swim or walking when the heat of the day has passed will reduce pitta. It is also possible to have too little of a particular dosha, but most problems and ailments are a result of a doshic increase rather than a decrease. Keeping your doshas in balance will not only help to promote your health generally, it will also counteract stress. This is because you will be acting in accordance with the laws of nature—and in some cases, those of simple common sense. If you are feeling tired because you have been partying all night (a vata state), you need to rest. If, however, you are tired because you are feeling bored and lethargic (a kapha state), the best thing you can do is go for a long run.

This is not to suggest, however, that the three doshas should be in an equal ratio to each other. Everyone is born with a completely individual doshic balance and it is this that forms your basic constitution, or prakriti. It is when one dosha is aggravated to such an extent that it upsets this inner balance that problems arise.

The aim of ayurveda is to overcome imbalances by means of diet or lifestyle changes and restore your natural harmony. The following pages will introduce you to the doshas in more detail. Once you have an understanding of the nature of ayurveda and the three doshas, you will be able to use the questionnaire in the following chapter to help you discover your own prakriti.

Keeping your **doshas in balance** will not only promote your health generally, it will also **counteract stress.**

Vata

Vata is the king dosha. It governs movement, and the other two doshas need vata because they cannot move or function on their own. If vata is kept in check, pitta and kapha will not go out of balance either. Because of its mobility, however, vata is also the most unstable dosha, the one most likely to go out of balance and, ultimately, to cause disease.

Vata elements
Ether and air

Vata in nature
The vata principle is best seen in wind and the currents of the oceans.

Vata qualities
Cold, dry, erratic, moving, lightweight, scattered, subtle, clear, rough, coarse, brittle and small

Vata functions
Movement, communication and travel

Physical characteristics
People whose dominant dosha is vata typically show physical characteristics of slightness, dryness and some irregularity or angularity. Vata is both the smallest and the tallest of the three doshas, as well as the thinnest, in terms of overall body frame, and people with this dominant dosha often find it difficult to put on weight. Vatas' skin and hair

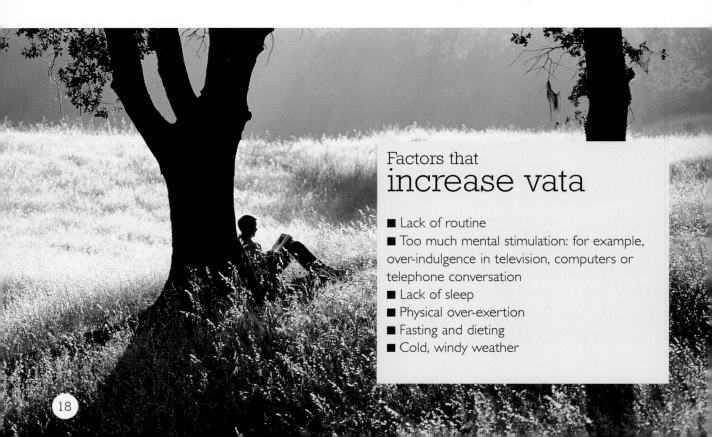

Factors that
increase vata

- Lack of routine
- Too much mental stimulation: for example, over-indulgence in television, computers or telephone conversation
- Lack of sleep
- Physical over-exertion
- Fasting and dieting
- Cold, windy weather

are usually dry and hair is also likely to be dark, thick and wiry, and often curly or wavy. Vatas usually have a thin and angular face with small, dull, brown or grey eyes, and a narrow nose and mouth. The teeth are often irregular. Vata babies are usually small. Vatas sweat very little and have light, restless sleep.

Locations of vata

According to ayurveda, each dosha has specific locations and functions within the body. Vata is located in five sites:

PRANA VATA
Brain, head, throat, heart, lungs
Prana vata controls breathing, reasoning, feeling and sensory perception.

UDANA VATA
Throat, lungs, navel
Udana vata governs the voice and energy.

SAMANA VATA
Stomach, intestines
Samana vata energizes pitta's power to digest food and governs peristalsis (see Apana vata).

APANA VATA
Colon (the seat of vata), bladder, rectum, sexual organs
Apana vata controls menstruation, elimination of excretory and sexual waste products.

VYANA VATA
Nervous system, skin, circulation of blood
Vyana vata governs the circulation, blood pressure and the sense of touch.

Vata's senses

Vata needs to be warmed and soothed through all the senses.

SOUND: Vatas needs silence, chanting or quiet, calming music.

TOUCH: Massage with warm sesame oil.

SIGHT: Bright, calming and warming natural colors—combinations of yellow, orange, green, blue and cream.

TASTE: Nourishing, rich, oily foods with plenty of sweet, salty and sour tastes and moderately spiced.

SMELL: Warm, sweet, calming fragrances, such as jasmine and lavender.

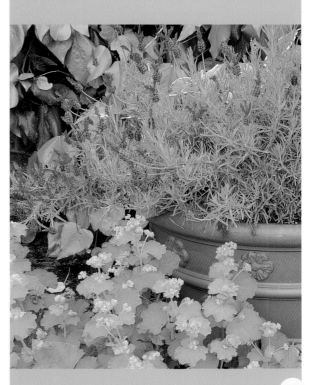

Mental, emotional and behavioral characteristics

Vata is the most active dosha, always on the move both physically and mentally. Vatas are full of ideas, often darting from one to another and eager to communicate them to others. Vatas have a good short-term memory and learn new things quickly. Conversely, their long-term memory is poor, with a tendency to forget things as quickly as they have been learnt. Vatas' energy comes in short, intense spurts, during which a lot may be accomplished, but energy supplies are quickly depleted and Vatas are more prone to nervous disorders than any other type. They have difficulty making decisions and often doubt their own abilities. The most likely type to worry, they can easily become hypochondriacs and need a lot of support. They are happy to talk about a problem, but find it difficult to take and sustain practical action to combat it. They often get so caught up in a problem that they cannot see it clearly, whatever advice they are given. It is better for them to achieve one practical change than talk about ten good intentions.

Vata is the most sensitive of the doshas. Badly affected by negative atmospheres, Vatas should remove themselves quickly. Ill at ease, they fidget and pace the floor. While they are very sensitive to their own needs, when out of balance they can sometimes be less aware of others'. Vatas should be approached gently, with calmness and sensitivity, as they are easily hurt.

Vatas are extremely enthusiastic and always excited by new ideas. They approach a new job, sport or relationship with great excitement, but, having unrealistic expectations, this seldom lasts and they are quickly frustrated. Vatas' creativity and imagination make them natural artists in all media and it is vital for them to express this creativity or it will leave them feeling frustrated and unfulfilled.

Vatas are friendly, generous and enthusiastic people, eager for pleasure and entertainment, bubbly and bright. They are great individualists, so don't make particularly good leaders or followers either. Trying to organize a group of Vatas is rather like herding squirrels. They are not particularly materialistic and tend not to accumulate possessions, while they treat money on an easy-come, easy-go basis.

To be in balance, Vatas need to express their emotions and creativity, release fear and anxiety, give and receive massage to warm the heart, and take up grounding activities such as gardening. In relationships, their ideal partner would have a strong kapha constitution, which will create a stable and serene atmosphere.

Vata times & seasons

During the course of every twenty-four hours, vata is at its peak during the afternoon, from 2 to 6, and again from 2 to 6 in the morning. Seasonally, vata's time is autumn and early winter, or at any time when the weather is cold, windy and dry. All of these times and conditions serve to aggravate and increase vata.

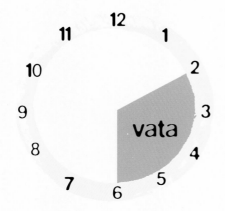

Talking to Vatas

Conversation with Vata people is likely to be disjointed, flitting from one subject to another, particularly when they are under pressure. When you talk to Vatas, you should always hold eye contact and talk softly and slowly—this will hold their attention, which may otherwise wander to something else. Vatas will often ask another question halfway through your answer to a first one. Don't expect direct, logical answers from Vatas but rather something like this:

Q: Where are the car keys?
V: In my wallet.
Q: Where is your wallet?
V: In my coat.
Q: Where is your coat?
V: In the car.

This can be quite funny when you understand the Vata makeup, but an out-of-balance, angry Pitta will be driven demented by it.

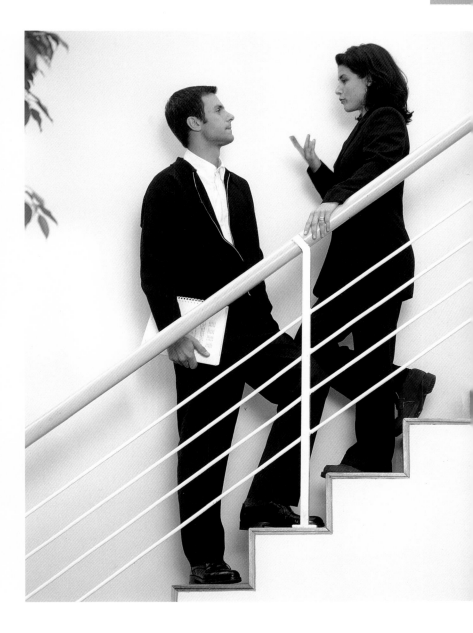

Vata in and out of balance

When vata is in balance, it is the dosha of enthusiasm, creativity and ideas: generous, artistic and free-thinking. When you have a vata imbalance, these positive qualities can be translated into anxiety, restlessness and fear. Physical symptoms of a vata imbalance include dry, rough skin, insomnia, joint problems, constipation, poor circulation with cold hands and feet, breathing difficulties, headaches, tinnitus, weight loss, flatulence, brittle nails and hair, menstrual cramps and PMS, and high blood pressure. Emotionally, you can be cold and aloof, selfish, over-sensitive, forgetful, vague, unrealistic, neurotic or melodramatic. You will probably become anxious, irrational and have low confidence, forgetting to eat properly (vital for a grounded Vata) and out of touch with your body.

21

Pitta

Pitta is the dosha of transformation. It governs the digestion and metabolism of food and the body's biochemical activities. Pitta is the intellectual of the doshas, with a precise mind that does not suffer fools gladly.

Pitta elements
Fire and water

Pitta in nature
Fire and the heat of the sun exemplify pitta in nature.

Pitta qualities
Hot, sharp, bright, liquid, slightly oily, sour and pungent

Pitta functions
All transformation and metabolism, particularly digestion, vision, comprehension, courage and complexion

Physical characteristics
People whose dominant dosha is pitta are typically fair-skinned, often with freckles, birthmarks or moles, and they have fine fair or red hair which often turns grey or falls out prematurely. They have

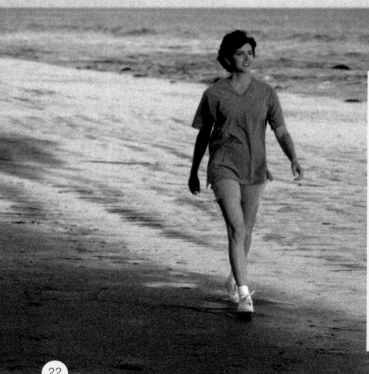

Factors that
increase pitta

- Heat—whether overheated rooms or too much sun
- Hunger, not eating regular meals, eating when upset or angry
- Competition
- Salt, spicy and sour foods
- Exercising during pitta time (10 A.M. – 2 P.M.)
- Alcohol
- Too much mental activity, unbalanced by physical activity

light-colored, intense eyes, usually blue or grey, occasionally hazel. They often have a heart-shaped face and a pointed nose and chin. They have a medium build with no strong tendency either to gain or to lose weight. They are fairly active and sweat profusely in hot weather. They will sleep soundly but for quite a short time and, being the dosha that governs digestion, they experience the fiercest hunger pangs.

Locations of pitta

According to ayurveda, each dosha has specific locations and functions within the body. Pitta is located in five sites:

PACHAKA PITTA
Stomach and small intestine

Pachaka pitta controls the digestion and absorption of food and its nutrients—this is the most important role of pitta in the body.

RANJAKA PITTA
Liver, spleen, red blood cells

Ranjaka pitta is responsible for the formation of red blood cells and the lymph, the fluid of the lymphatic system, the basis of the body's immune system.

SADHAKA PITTA
Heart

According to ayurveda, the heart is the seat of consciousness and so sadhaka pitta governs the emotions, intelligence and memory.

ALOCHAKA PITTA
Eyes

Alochaka pitta is responsible for sight.

BHRAJAKA PITTA
Skin

Bhrajaka pitta governs skin metabolism and color.

Pitta's senses

Pitta needs to be cooled and calmed through all the senses.

SOUND: Cooling, soft, calm music such as the flute, the sound of the sea, waterfalls, running water.

TOUCH: Moderate pressure massage with coconut oil.

SIGHT: Cooling colors, such as blues, greens and cream.

TASTE: Cooling herbs and spices, such as cumin, turmeric, fennel and aniseed. Sweet, bitter and astringent tastes.

SMELL: Cool, sweet smells, such as sandalwood, rose and jasmine.

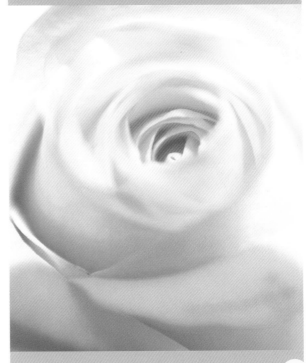

Mental, emotional and behavioral characteristics

Pitta is the most organized and ambitious of the doshas, meticulous at forward-planning as well as following the plans through to their conclusion. They are the most intellectual of the doshas, logical and precise, with good concentration and memory and an ability to argue their case well and persuasively. Pittas make excellent public speakers. Natural skeptics, Pittas never shy away from challenging anything or anybody. They have a love of

Pitta times & seasons

During the course of every twenty-four hours, pitta is at its peak during the middle of the day, from 10 to 2, and again from 10 to 2 in the night. Seasonally, pitta's time is the mid to late summer, or at any time when the weather is hot, and especially if it is humid too. All of these times and conditions serve to aggravate and increase pitta.

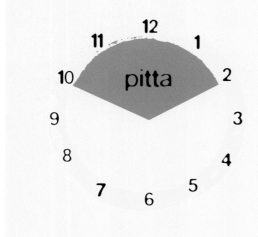

order and authority and are impressed with status and credentials.

They are confident, brave and alert, with a natural thirst for knowledge. Humor is very important to Pitta types and it is an instant barometer to mood—they need to laugh to prevent them becoming too intense, while loss of sense of humor should be a warning indicator. Pittas make loyal, warm-hearted and helpful friends, but cruel and unforgiving enemies, and, because of their own inherent self-discipline, they can be very self-righteous if they feel others don't measure up. They shouldn't expect so much and put themselves under such pressure. Being perfectionists, they can become pedantic when out of balance and follow regimes and instructions rigidly to the letter—there is a definite militaristic bent to their temperament. They should beware of developing a "hang 'em and flog 'em" attitude! Anyone or anything that is vague or indecisive will drive Pittas to distraction. In fact, living with a Pitta can be very trying as they honestly believe they are always right. A partner who can keep calm at all times is ideal for Pitta types.

To be in balance, it is vital for Pittas to learn to look at all points of view in a balanced way and not simply to stick rigidly to their own opinions. Tact and diplomacy are the qualities they most need to acquire. In relationships Pittas should watch out for jealousy and controlling behavior. They are naturally passionate, but they must take care that they are not so intense that they consume and burn out their partner. Anger and aggression should be released and they should lighten up—spending time playing with young children (to promote innocence and a warm heart) is effective, and finding things that make them laugh.

Pitta in and out of balance

When pitta is in balance, it is the dosha of confidence, courage and intelligence. When you have a pitta imbalance, however, these positive qualities

Talking to Pittas

Pittas' intense focus and eye for detail make them lucid thinkers and talkers and often inspiring public speakers. Being so focussed themselves, they expect a clear, precise answer and waffling enrages them. It is a good idea to be direct and factual when talking to Pittas, but with a warm tone and a smiling face as Pittas can easily become confrontational. If you are friendly and efficient you can generally calm down overheated Pittas, but if you get angry too, their tempers will spiral out of control. Pittas do not back down. Pittas are often not aware that people think their blunt-talking and passionate stare are aggressive as they feel they are just being direct and to the point.

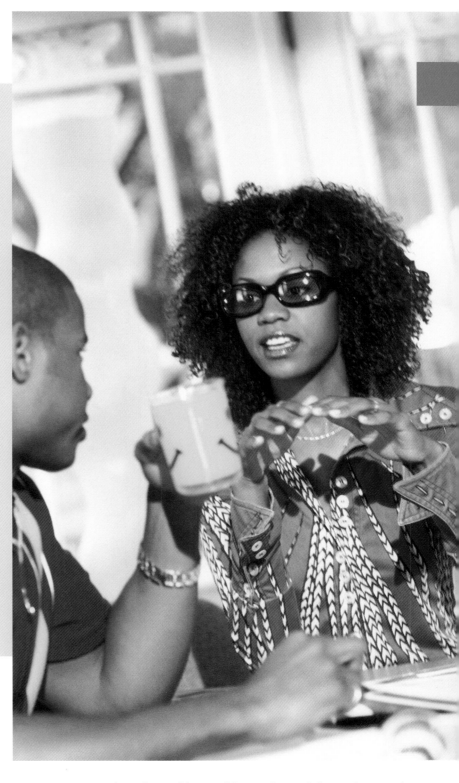

can be translated into irritability, stubbornness and impatience, aggression and a tendency to be judgmental and critical. Physical symptoms of a pitta imbalance include indigestion, diarrhea, heartburn, ulcers, hyperacidity, anemia and other blood disorders, jaundice, skin problems (especially rashes and acne), eye problems (especially bloodshot eyes) and heart disease.

Kapha

Kapha is the strongest dosha—with a strength that is both physical and psychological. It is also the most stable of the doshas, and the least likely to go out of balance and bring about disease. Kapha is slow to rouse to extremes of emotion or activity, but the most able to sustain and endure.

Kapha elements
Earth and water

Kapha in nature
Kapha gives an underlying structure to the natural world, its rocks, mountains and earth.

Kapha qualities
Heavy, slow, cold, large, oily, sweet, soft and stable

Kapha functions
Structure, stamina and lubrication

Physical characteristics
People whose dominant dosha is kapha are usually short with a large frame and chest and have obvious physical strength. Kaphas put on weight easily and find it hard to lose it again. Kaphas' skin is usually pale and oily, while their hair is likely

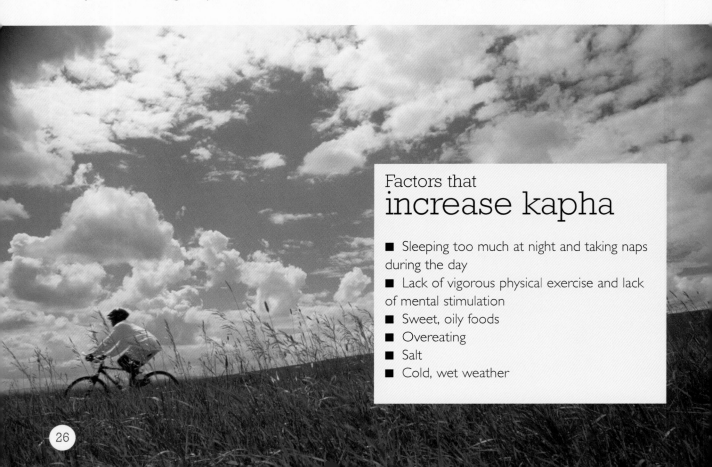

Factors that
increase kapha

- Sleeping too much at night and taking naps during the day
- Lack of vigorous physical exercise and lack of mental stimulation
- Sweet, oily foods
- Overeating
- Salt
- Cold, wet weather

to be thick, wavy and dark. Kaphas have a good bone structure and their faces are often large and round, with a thick-set neck, large, blue or brown eyes, and a large nose and mouth. The teeth are often small and white. Kapha babies are usually heavy. Kaphas sweat moderately once stimulated and sleep very deeply and more than the other doshas.

Locations of kapha

According to ayurveda, each dosha has specific locations and functions within the body. Kapha is located in five sites:

KLEDAKA KAPHA
Stomach

Kledaka kapha moistens and initiates the digestion of food.

AVALAMBAKA KAPHA
Chest, heart, lungs

Avalambaka kapha supports the heart and chest.

BODHAKA KAPHA
Tongue, throat

Bodhaka kapha moistens the tongue, secretes mucus in the throat and recognizes taste.

TARPAKA KAPHA
Head

Tarpaka kapha maintains spinal fluid, moistens the nose, mouth and eyes, and supports the brain and sensory organs.

SHLESHAKA KAPHA
Joints

Shleshaka kapha lubricates the joints throughout the body.

Kapha's senses

Stimulation is the key to kapha's senses being in balance.

SOUND: Loud, fast music—get dancing!

TOUCH: Firm, deep massage using raw silk gloves or a dry herbalized paste (see pages 132 and 133).

SIGHT: Loud, bright, tropical colors. Strong reds, oranges, yellows and gold.

TASTE: Pungent, bitter, astringent flavors. Use black pepper, cloves, cinnamon and powdered ginger.

SMELL: Pungent fragrances, such as eucalyptus, cedar, rosemary, juniper and camphor. Olbas oil is a combination of kapha oils and is a great inhalant or muscle rub.

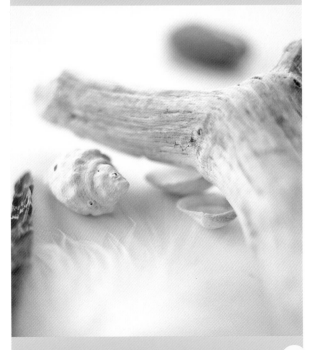

Mental, emotional and behavioral characteristics

Kapha is the most stable of the three doshas: patient, grounded and caring. Kapha types are faithful and supportive, compassionate and affectionate. Sometimes slow to learn, Kaphas' long-term memories are excellent. Kaphas move and talk slowly, but have great reserves of energy and stamina when needed. Honorable and gentle, Kaphas are patient and slow to anger, but equally slow to calm down.

Kapha times & seasons

During the course of every twenty-four hours, kapha is at its peak during the morning, from 6 to 10, and again from 6 to 10 in the evening. Seasonally, kapha's time is the late winter and early spring, and sometimes early summer, or at any time when the weather is cold, wet, dull and still. All of these times and conditions serve to aggravate and increase kapha.

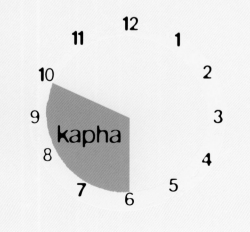

Kapha is the most sentimental and romantic of the three types and Kapha people are very tactile—they love to cuddle and feel at ease with someone else. Out of balance, however, they can become clinging and possessive and overly dependent on others. Their desire to keep everything safe and familiar can, in the same circumstances, lead to controlling behavior in the form of emotional blackmail. The same impulse, in the home, makes them an inveterate hoarder.

Kaphas hate any kind of change. They genuinely cannot see the point and prefer it if everything is always done in the way they know best. This is partly due to their love of the familiar and partly to do with their feeling that they don't adapt well to change. Ironically, it is change that Kaphas need at a fairly constant rate, to keep them from feeling dull and bored. This boredom results not only in undesirable emotional behavior but also in overeating, physical inactivity and weight gain. Comfort-eating is a typically out-of-balance Kapha trait.

Kaphas should aim to become more independent. They should clear out their house, mind and emotions and they will actually feel more content, even physically lighter, although such activity does go against the grain. Kaphas need to exercise vigorously and regularly, not eat or sleep too much—or lie around in bed or in front of the television—and they should also surround themselves with bright colors and stimulating ideas and people. It may sound like a lot to cope with, but it makes Kaphas much more fulfilled and at peace.

Kapha in and out of balance

When kapha is in balance, it is the most centered and contented of the doshas. When you have a kapha imbalance, however, these positive qualities can change to their negative opposites, making you lazy and dull, greedy or possessive. Physical symptoms of a kapha imbalance include obesity, heart disease, back and joint problems, asthma, sinus problems, congestion and lethargy.

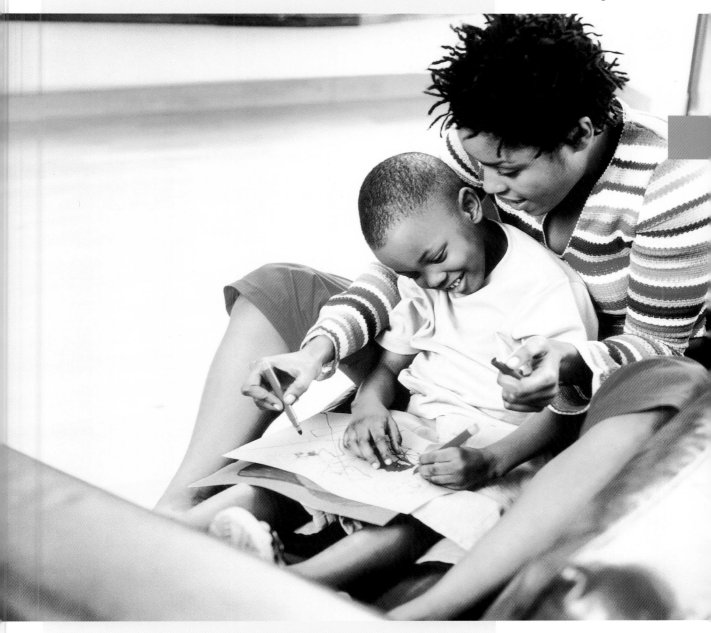

Talking to Kaphas

Kaphas speak slowly and carefully with deep, melodic voices, and, being quiet by nature, are happy to let others take the spotlight. When you talk to a Kapha, you will get the best response if you are lively and enthusiastic—this lifts their spirits. Kaphas are the best listeners and, having a soft heart, the perfect shoulder to cry on.

Chapter two

Discovering your dosha

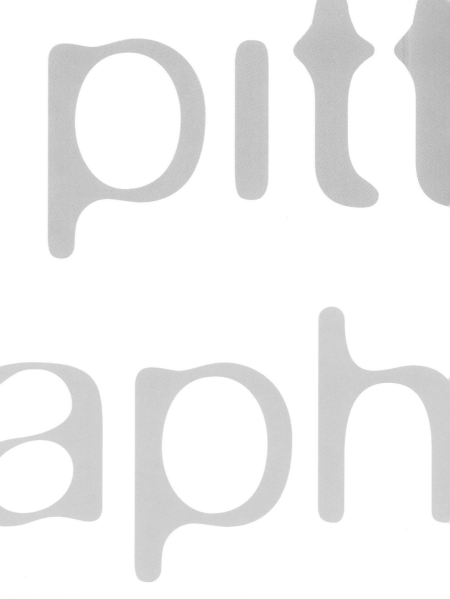

The key to unlocking the door to ayurvedic health is your dosha. Your dosha defines your type—both of body and of mind—in much the same way as the humors were used in medieval times, each being identified with an underlying element. There are three doshas—vata (air and ether), pitta (fire and water) and kapha (earth and water). If you're predominantly vata, you're likely to be thin, quick-thinking and restless; pittas have quick tempers and a tendency to digestive disorders; and kaphas are slower both physically and temperamentally with a tendency to gain weight.

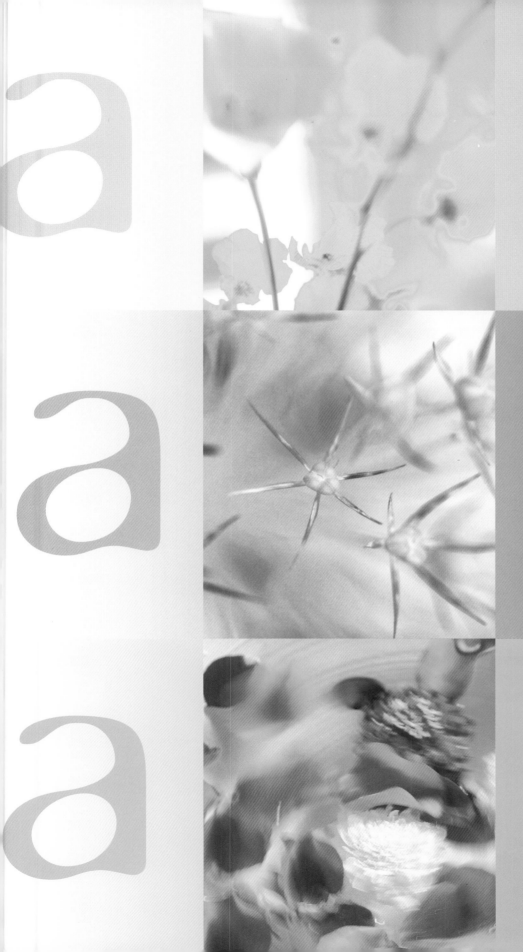

Vata people

Temperament: enthusiastic, quick-thinking, restless, sensitive

Characteristics: dark-skinned, the smallest or tallest of the doshas, the thinnest in terms of body frame

Pitta people

Temperament: perfectionist, ambitious, confident and quick-tempered

Characteristics: fair-skinned, light-colored eyes, medium build

Kapha people

Temperament: patient, caring, supportive and compassionate

Characteristics: pale-skinned, large-framed, strong

Questionnaire

The questionnaire is split into three sections, the first two requiring both A and B answers. Your answers to the A questions tell you your dominant dosha, while the B questions indicate any current imbalance. It is important to keep the tally of each section and of the A and B questions separate. Use the charts on page 37 to help you keep track of your answers.

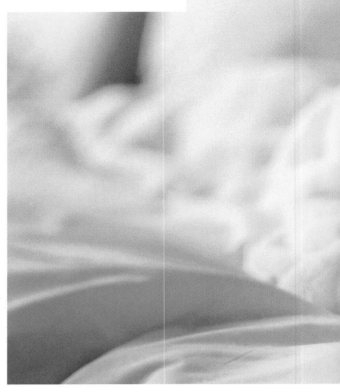

Everybody is made up of a combination of the three doshas. However, there is usually a dominant one and once you know what this is you can set about correcting any imbalances you may have, as well as adapting everything from your diet to your garden to create a healthier, happier lifestyle. Besides having one leading and one secondary dosha, you may also have a doshic imbalance—and this can sometimes be the third dosha! Unraveling all of this can be quite complicated and it is vital to get a true picture if you are going to make ayurveda work for you.

An ayurvedic health practitioner who is experienced at identifying doshas can do this by taking your pulses. Ayurvedic pulse-taking is quite different than the Western kind and an altogether longer process, taking several minutes. The pulse is felt at different pressures and in different places to give a complete picture of your constitution and imbalances.

You can also use the following questionnaire, based on the one used at the European Ayurveda spa. It has been carefully prepared to give an accurate reading of both your principal dosha and any imbalance you may have—a common problem with most ayurvedic questionnaires where the two tend to be muddled. The questionnaire is divided into three main parts: the body, the mind and emotions, and, because it is so central to assessing your constitution, the digestion. Keep the A and B answers and the scores for each section separately.

The first part (A) of each question gives your body type, while the second part (B) identifies any imbalance. In the digestion section there are no Bs, and there is also no B in other parts of the questionnaire where it does not apply.

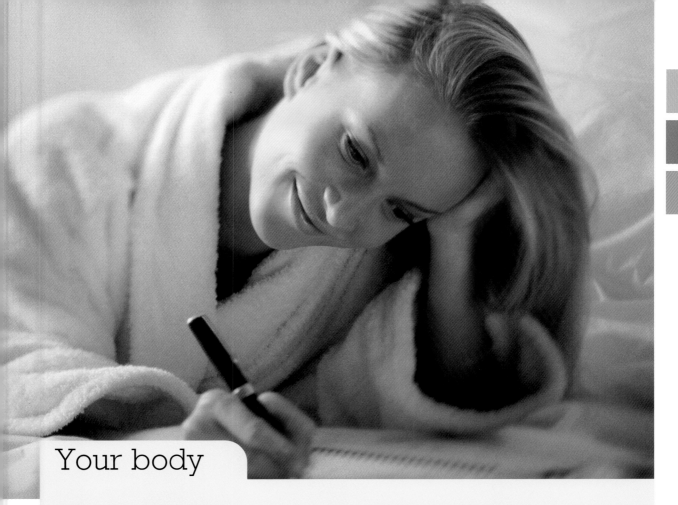

Your body

1A How would you describe your skin?
Dry, rough, cold to touch   V
Fair, soft, warm to touch   P
Pale, cold, clammy, oily   K

1B Have you experienced any of these skin problems recently?
Very dry skin with rough patches   V
Heat rashes, spots   P
Excessive oiliness   K

2A How would you describe your hair?
Dry, coarse, brittle, fine to medium   V
Fine, fair or reddish   P
Thick, oily, lustrous   K

2B Have you noticed any of these hair problems recently?
Brittle, with split ends   V
Thinning, graying, balding   P
Excessive oiliness   K

3 What is your body size and frame?
Lean, thin, often quite tall   V
Medium height/build, good muscle tone   P
Plump, stocky, large chest, often short   K

4A In general, what is your weight?
Light, finding it hard to gain weight   V
Medium, gaining and losing weight easily   P
Heavy, finding it hard to lose weight   K

4B What is your recent weight?
Underweight   V
Fluctuating weight   P
Overweight   K

5A What is your tolerance to heat?

High, enjoying heat `V`

Poor, preferring moderate to cool `P`
High, preferring hot, dry weather `K`

5B In heat, how much do your perspire?

Minimally `V`

Freely, especially during exercise `P`
Clammy, not free-flowing `K`

6A What is your normal body temperature throughout the year?

Low, with cold hands and feet `V`
High, feeling warm or hot `P`
Low, body feels cold `K`

6B How has your body temperature affected you recently?

Always cold, feeling below par `V`
When hot, feeling irritated or angry `P`
Cold, lethargic physically and mentally `K`

7A Which type of weather do you prefer?

Hot and humid, sunny and tropical `V`
Moderate to cool `P`
Hot and dry, sunny and windy `K`

7B Which type of weather do you find most uncomfortable?

Cold, windy, dry `V`
Heat, especially when sitting in sun `P`
Cold, damp `K`

8A How well do you sleep generally?

Light, disturbed sleep for 5 to 6 hours `V`
Fairly sound, 6 to 8 hours `P`
Heavy, deep prolonged sleep,
8 hours or more `K`

8B How well have you been sleeping recently?

Waking between 2 A.M. and 6 A.M. `V`
Problems getting to sleep, but then a
sound sleep `P`
Sleeping over 10 hours, hard to wake up `K`

9A How would you describe your energy levels?

Short bursts of energy, low endurance,
small reserves `V`
Moderate endurance, good reserves `P`
Good stamina, strong, large reserves `K`

9B What is your recent experience?

Feeling exhausted, low reserves `V`
Feeling tired, but able to recover quickly `P`
Constant energy, good reserves `K`

10A In general, how are your physical movements best described?

Quick-moving, erratic, hyperactive `V`
Moderately active, motivated, purposeful `P`
Slow, steady, graceful movements `K`

10B What is your recent experience?

Feeling clumsy, uncoordinated `V`
Movements feel strident, regimented `P`
Feeling lethargic, lackluster `K`

Your mind & emotions

1A Describe your usual mental state:
A quick mind and a restless imagination V
Intellectual, well organized and efficient,
perfectionist P
Steady, calm, not easily disturbed K

1B Have you experienced any of the
following recently?
Feeling ungrounded, disconnected V
Impatience, irritability, anger P
Feeling slow, dull, uninspired K

2A Would you describe your mental attitude
and approach to life as:
Creative, expressive, unbounded V
Determined, goal-oriented, passionate P
Contented, calm, methodical K

2B Have you recently felt any of the following?
Anxious, indecisive, confused V
Pedantic, critical, fanatical P
Over-dependent, lethargic, resistant to
change K

3A How would you describe your memory?
Quick to retain information initially,
quick to forget V
Good general memory, clear intellect P
Slow to retain at first, good long-term
memory K

3B Have you recently experienced any of
the following?
Forgetfulness, difficulty focussing and
concentrating V
Focussing only on the negative P
Slow, labored attempts to retain
information, lacking in clarity K

4A What is your normal response to stress?
Anxious, fearful V
Confrontational, forceful P
Quiet, introverted K

4B What has been your recent reaction
to stress?
Tearful, with irrational fears V
Aggressive, hot-tempered P
Tendency to withdraw and bury your
head in the sand K

5 How would you describe your convictions
and beliefs?
Changeable, rebellious V
Strongly held P
Constant, conservative K

6A How would you describe your approach
to life?
Erratic, unplanned, a free spirit V
Ambitious, carefully planned, an achiever P
Safe, steady, regular, resistant to change K

6B How have you felt recently?
Chaotic, indecisive V
Over-ambitious, discontented, forcing
the pace P
Stuck in a rut, procrastinating K

7A Which positive attributes describe you best?
Enthusiastic, creative, adaptable   V
Courageous, humorous, keen intellect   P
Loyal, dependable, forgiving   K

7B When you feel out of balance, do you experience the following?
Feelings of isolation, life loses its beauty   V
Loss of humor   P
You feel dull, lifeless   K

8A On a good day, how do you feel?
Secure, grounded, settled   V
Confident, friendly, contented   P
Warm-hearted, loving, active   K

8B When you are upset, how do you feel?
Cold, distant   V
Jealous, controlling   P
Possessive, clinging   K

Your digestion

1 How is your digestion and appetite normally?
Irregular and erratic   V
Sharp and strong, you feel uncomfortable missing meals   P
Slow and weak, you miss meals easily   K

2 Which of these do you most commonly experience after eating?
Bloating, wind, feeling toxic   V
Heartburn, stomach acid, a sour feeling   P
Heaviness, sluggishness   K

3 How would you normally describe your bowel movements?
Irregular   V
Regular, more than once a day   P
Slow but regular   K

4 Do you experience any of the following?
Constipation   V
Loose stools, diarrhea   P
Heavy, dense stools   K

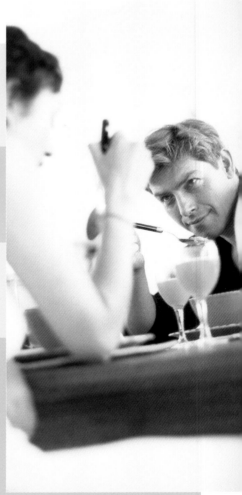

Use these charts to work out your own doshic makeup. Color in one block for each answer you give. So, if you scored six Vs and four Ps in the Your Body A questions, then you will have colored in the first six segments of the V column and the first four segments of the P column.

Your body

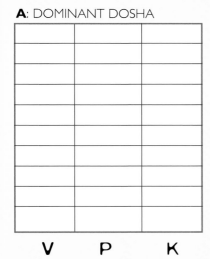

A: DOMINANT DOSHA

V　　　P　　　K

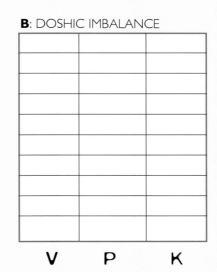

B: DOSHIC IMBALANCE

V　　　P　　　K

Analysis
The answers to these questions give you your dominant body type and indicate any imbalances you may have. Use the information on pages 38–9 to help you interpret your score.

Your mind & emotions

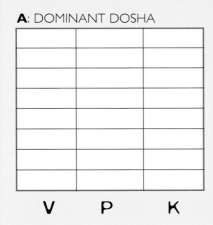

A: DOMINANT DOSHA

V　　　P　　　K

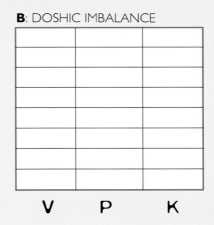

B: DOSHIC IMBALANCE

V　　　P　　　K

Analysis
The answers to these questions give you a greater understanding of how you think and feel and indicate any imbalances you may have. Use the information on pages 38–9 to help you interpret your score.

Your digestion

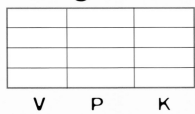

V　　　P　　　K

Analysis
The answers to these questions give you your digestive type. Use the information on pages 38–9 to help you decide on the diet plan for your digestive type.

Interpreting the questionnaire

Now that you have answered the questionnaire and tallied up your answers, you need to know how to interpret the information you have.

The two first sections, the Body questionnaire and the Mind & Emotions questionnaire, give you your predominant body type (part As) and therefore a greater understanding of the forces that make up how you think and feel. They also indicate any imbalances (part Bs) you may have. To create a sense of harmony and well-being, it is important to pacify your imbalance using the appropriate daily routine (see pages 108–17). So if, for instance, you mostly get P answers for part A but some V answers too, your body type is pitta/vata. If you get mostly V answers for the B questions you have a vata imbalance. You should therefore follow the vata daily routine (pages 108–10) until the vata imbalance has been corrected. Then you follow the general guidelines for your principal dosha, in this case the pitta daily routine (pages 112–15). Make sure you exercise too, according to the recommendations given for your principal dosha.

The digestion section gives you your diet plan. Whatever your body type, follow the diet plan for your digestive type, as the Digestion questionnaire reveals. Don't follow the diet plan for your body type unless it happens to be the same as your digestive type.

Although this questionnaire will help guide you to particular sections suited to you, it is important to read the other sections because, as mentioned, most people do find they are a mixture of doshas although one or two are often dominant. By looking at all the sections you will learn to identify some aspects of other doshas which are relevant to you, you will learn to understand yourself and, by the process of self-referral, realize what puts you in and out of balance.

Chapter by chapter, this book will help you to form a complete picture of yourself. By looking at the changing seasons and cycles which affect us all (Chapter 3), your diet (Chapter 4) and exercise regime (Chapter 5), followed by a recommended daily routine (Chapter 5), you will then be able to consider how meditation (Chapter 6), massage (Chapter 7) and designing your environment (Chapter 8) all impact on your well-being.

Dealing with stress

The overriding aim of ayurveda, as we have seen, is to achieve harmony in life so that your own inner balance effectively eradicates potential stress and illness. Living in the modern world, it may seem surprising that this ancient body of knowledge is relevant to and successful at dealing with stress—something many of us regard as a contemporary phenomenon. However, stress and the sense of not being at ease have always led, as medical research increasingly reveals, all too easily to disease.

There are, though, many ways of looking at stress. Most commonly, it is seen as a mental or emotional pressure that the world outside inflicts on us—it might be office politics, relationship problems or getting stuck in traffic when you're in a hurry. You can also heap stress upon yourself by not getting enough sleep, eating the wrong kinds of food or wearing yourself out with an exhausting form of exercise. The stress in this case is caused by putting yourself under a physical strain. However, according to the principles of ayurveda—and indeed those of many modern stress-management techniques—there is no tangible division between mind and body and so stress to either body or mind will flow quite naturally from one to the other.

The importance of the daily routines

Because we are so used to taking a pill as a cure for just about any ailment we have, we are also inclined to continue loading yet more stresses and strains on to our bodies and minds. Instead of seeing constant headaches or digestive problems as a warning that something is going wrong, we seek out an over-the-counter medicine—a painkiller, a laxative, an antacid—to hold things at bay and carry on regardless. The cycle continues until the problem is sufficiently serious to make us take notice.

Ayurveda takes a very different approach to health and stress management. It regards both illness and stress as signs that you are not in a state of harmony, either within yourself or with the world around you, and its aim is to find a way to restore that missing harmony. Much of this harmony comes from understanding who you are—your prakriti—and, armed with that knowledge, how to achieve both health and happiness.

How does this work? Each dosha, as we have seen, has very particular characteristics and, if you struggle against the prevailing currents of your own physiology, you are only too likely to become ill or stressed. If, for instance, you have a predominantly pitta constitution, you must have regular meals. If you skip lunch, you will find your afternoon turns into a nightmare—you can't concentrate, you become irritable and you achieve very little. If you eat a satisfying meal in the middle of the day, your

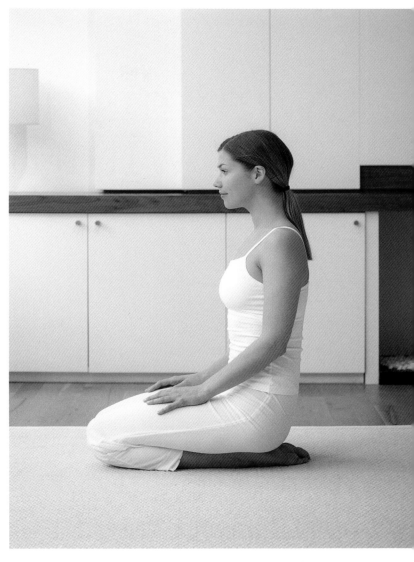

afternoon will be transformed. On the other hand, if you're mostly kapha, indulging in a nap will not make you feel rested, it will just make you feel lethargic and listless for the entire day. Kapha types will be much more energized and enthusiastic about life by making an early start and taking vigorous exercise in the morning.

While there are certain universal ayurvedic rules for living a healthy and contented life, there are some that apply to each dosha individually. These relate in part to the dominant bodily and mental functions of each dosha and also to the rhythm of the day as it passes through the cycle of the three doshas twice every twenty-four hours—this is explained in greater depth on pages 42–5.

Chapter three

Swimming
with the tide

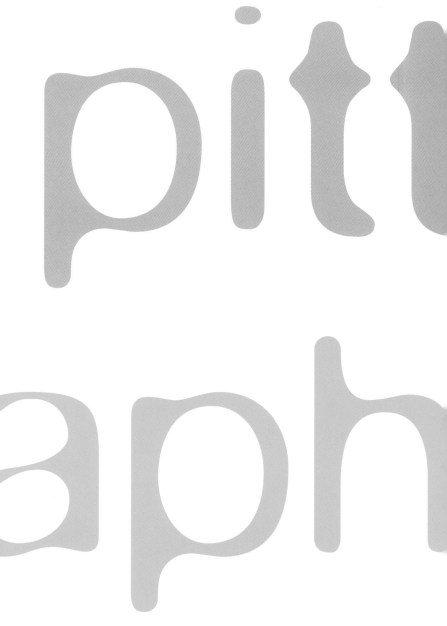

The doshas do not just apply to people, they relate to everything around us. They have their own times of day and seasons of the year and we experience their subtle changes through all areas of our lives. Understanding these rhythms, we can incorporate them into our lives, avoiding doing the right thing at the wrong time and reinforcing the effects of whatever we want to achieve—from getting fit to having a good night's sleep. As you become more aware of the doshic cycles, you will find you are less stressed. You will also become more at ease, both within yourself and with the world.

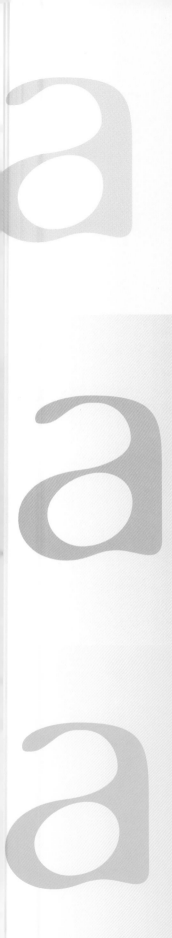

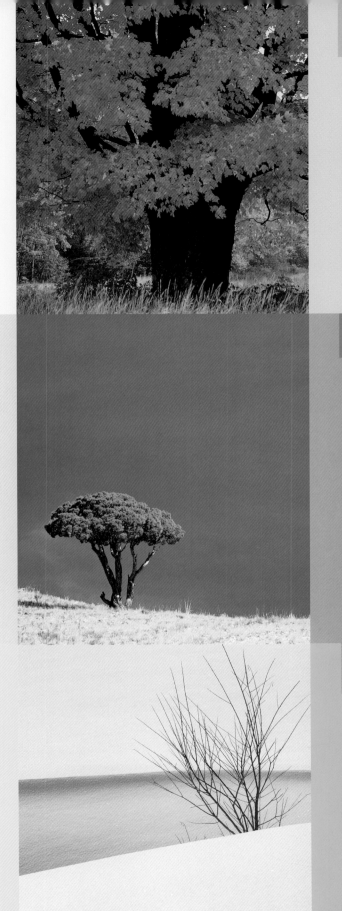

Vata

Season:
autumn and early
winter

Weather:
cold, dry, windy
weather

Pitta

Season:
mid and late
summer

Weather:
hot, humid weather

Kapha

Season:
late winter and
spring, and some-
times (depending
on local climate)
early summer

Weather:
cold, wet, dull,
still weather

The doshic clock

Every twenty-four hours, we travel through two doshic cycles. Vata runs from 2 to 6 in the morning, then again in the afternoons from 2 to 6. Pitta time is from 10 to 2 in the middle of the day and from 10 to 2 at night. Kapha time begins in the early morning from 6 to 10 and returns in the evening from 6 to 10.

The natural day

The day has its own natural rhythms and the closer we can follow them, the happier, healthier and less stressed we will feel. The further we stray from them, the more serious the repercussions for our health and well-being. Just think of the effects of jet-lag on both mind and body and the disorientation of people who work irregular shifts.

However, very few of us do follow the natural rhythms of the day, as our lives have strayed further and further from them, especially over the last century, when electricity revolutionized everyone's waking and sleeping habits. Our ancestors' lives were governed by nature. They would wake when it was light and go to sleep when it was dark. They didn't have much of an alternative, but nowadays we do. As a result, most of us are at least moving our day back by a couple of hours, getting up and going to bed later, and in some cases our waking and sleeping patterns are much more distorted than that. People stay up all night cramming for exams, working the night shift or partying. According to ayurveda, the closer you can keep to the day's own rhythms—ideally, up by 6 A.M. and in bed by 10 P.M.—the better you will feel. When you disrupt those patterns you need to compensate, pacifying the doshas you aggravate. The underlying reason for this is not simply due to natural light however.

The early morning is vata time. So if you wake up early, your entire day will have vata qualities—you will feel energetic, enthusiastic and alert. Conversely, the later you wake up, the more you get into kapha time and this again will affect your whole day, making you feel sluggish and lethargic. At night, ayurveda recommends going to bed by 10 P.M., while you are still in kapha time. During kapha time, you are likelier to fall into a deeper sleep from which you will wake feeling more refreshed. After kapha comes pitta time—the point at which you will get your second wind. Going to bed late, you will find it much harder to get into a sound sleep and you will tend to wake up next day still feeling tired. Having said this, no one can be expected to live out of step with the world around them—you would have a pretty short night out if you had to be back before 10 P.M. However, on those nights when you can go to bed early, it is worth looking at how it makes you feel the next day. If you have more energy and you feel more rested, you know that early nights and mornings are going to benefit you whenever you can get them. By incorporating them into your routine whenever you can, you will have grasped the first self-referral principle: no one knows your physiology as well as you do, so do whatever you know makes you feel better.

The importance of mealtimes

The ayurvedic understanding of the day's rhythms goes much further, though, than simply dividing it into sleeping and waking times. Because there are two revolutions of the doshas every twenty-four hours, it teaches that particular activities are appropriate at different times of the day, and nowhere is this more important than the times of your meals. Pitta is the dosha that governs your metabolism, in particular the processes of digestion and the absorption of nutrients from food.

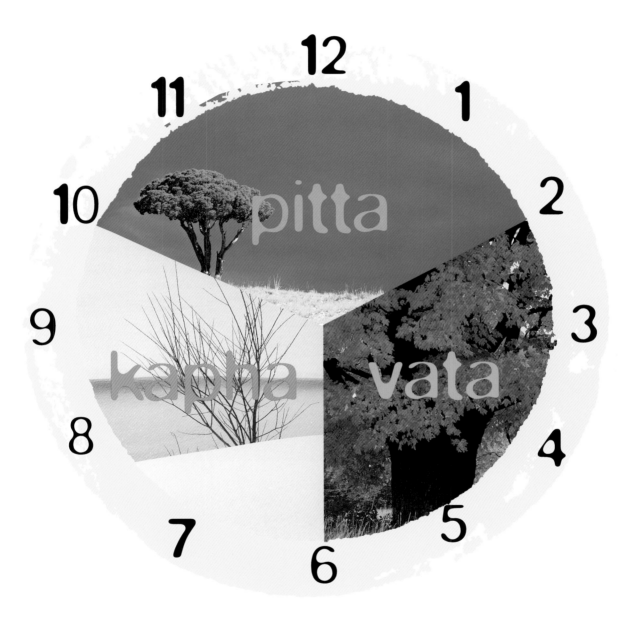

The doshic clock divides the day into six periods.
Vata time: 2 A.M. to 6 A.M. and 2 P.M. to 6 P.M.
Pitta time: 10 A.M. to 2 P.M. and 10 P.M. to 2 A.M.
Kapha time: 6 A.M. to 10 A.M. and 6 P.M. to 10 P.M.

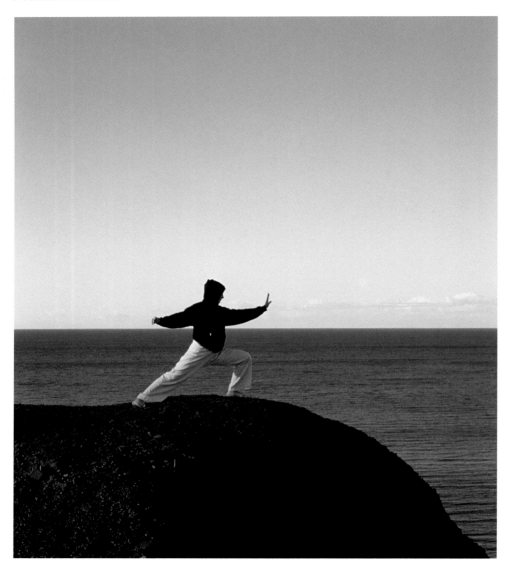

Ideally, then, you should eat the main meal of the day right in the middle of pitta time, around noon. In the evening, it is kapha time and your digestion is at its weakest. Meals eaten in the evening are not metabolized as well as they are in the day, and the later in the evening they are eaten—the further into kapha time—the more sluggish the digestive process becomes. It is better to eat a lighter, more easily digested meal in the evenings—preferably before 7 P.M.—avoiding fatty, sugary foods and also red meat. This not only allows your food to be digested before you go to bed, thus improving the quality of your sleep, it also enables pitta to focus on its metabolizing processes of cellular repair and renewal during the night, rather than simply digesting food. This eating pattern is particularly relevant to anyone who wants to lose weight – fatty or sugary foods eaten late in the evening are more likely to be stored as fat by the body.

Maximizing the benefits of exercise

It is during the kapha times of day that the body is at its strongest and has the most stamina, so this is the ideal time to take exercise. The morning (from 6 A.M. to 9 A.M.) is the best time of all, whatever your individual doshic makeup. Exercising at this time is both energizing and settling. It invigorates you, shaking off the last vestiges of sleep, and it is simultaneously grounding, giving a physical basis for your energies before you get swept up by the stresses of the day. Nowadays, when the vast majority of us work sitting at a desk, it is more important than ever to balance this sedentary existence with physical activity. And this is not just for the benefit of our heart or muscle tone. Exercise is mentally and emotionally grounding too and creates a platform of calm on which we can structure the rest of the day—particularly crucial for Vata and Pitta types.

The second kapha phase of the day is another good time to exercise, though it should be the first part of the cycle, from 6 P.M. to 8 P.M., as too much exercise too late in the day will be too invigorating for the physiology when it should be settling down, ready for sleep. Exercising too late will also take you dangerously close to pitta time, when you are more likely to push yourself too hard and risk injury. The middle of the day is the worst time to exercise. Skipping lunch to go to the gym will aggravate pitta so that, instead of making you feel invigorated and settled, you are more likely to be aggressive and irritable. And after 2 P.M. you are into vata time. It peaks between 3 and 4, when your energy tends to dip and you are physically at your weakest.

The cycle of the year

Just as the day moves through the doshas, an entire year has its own doshic pattern, with vata, pitta and kapha each having its own season. In traditional ayurveda, the seasons naturally relate to those of India and include a rainy season and a dry winter period as well as the wet one it shares with the West. In European ayurveda, the doshic seasons are adjusted to the different climatic conditions of the West. Each of these doshic seasons has a climate that increases the qualities of that dosha.

However, in many Western countries, the seasons are not as clearly defined as they are in the East—one season merges gradually into another and unseasonable weather conditions occur with increasing regularity. So summer, for instance, is—unfortunately—not necessarily hot, dry and sunny. It can all too often be wet or chilly instead. In this case, it is a kapha rather than a pitta day and kapha effects will apply. It is more helpful, then, to look at times of year and types of weather together.

VATA
autumn and early winter—cold, dry, windy weather

PITTA
mid and late summer—hot, humid weather

KAPHA
late winter and spring, and sometimes (depending on local climate) early summer—cold, wet, dull, still weather

The vata-aggravating season

During each of the doshic seasons or weather conditions, the prevailing dosha increases. Vata prefers hot, humid, still weather and so in the cold, dry, windy weather of the vata season, vata is aggravated and predominantly Vata people are the most unsettled by this—though vata increases for everyone at this time. This is when people are most at risk from vata ailments, such as colds, sore throats and respiratory infections, chapped lips and dry skin. It can also cause vata disturbances of the mind, such as irrational fears, forgetfulness, insomnia and anxiety.

In the vata season, excess vata can be pacified by keeping warm and by eating and drinking warm food and drinks—cold and especially icy drinks will only aggravate the situation.

The pitta-aggravating season

Pitta types prefer cool weather, so when the season is itself pitta you need to turn down the heat! This is particularly important for Pitta types, but it is relevant for everyone. In dietary terms, you should favor cold and cooling foods and drinks over hot, salty, sour and spicy ones, and eat less of all of them than you would in the winter. In fact, this is a natural urge for most people, who instinctively eat less but drink more in hot weather.

Very vigorous exercise is not advisable in hot weather—and everyone will naturally be sweatier than usual—but swimming is beneficial because of the cooling effect of water and Pittas will benefit, too, from cooling showers. Everyone is now aware of the dangers of the sun and skin cancer, so sunbathing or exposure to the sun without sufficient protection should always be avoided. Pitta types should also keep out of hot environments in the summer—a hot kitchen on a scorching summer day is guaranteed to make Pittas' tempers boil over. Conversely, walking in the evening, especially by water, in woodland and in moonlight, soothes and

calms further. The head and ears particularly need to be wrapped up in windy weather. A daily sesame oil massage (see pages 134–7) is very settling. Yoga and meditation are helpful, as is the company of trusted friends.

The kapha-aggravating season

The weather that suits Kapha people best is hot and dry. The cold, wet, dull weather that characterizes kapha gives rise to kapha ailments based on forms of congestion, such as coughs, colds and sinusitis, as well as joint problems and rheumatism. To counteract cold, damp, mucus-forming kapha, eat plenty of spicy, bitter and astringent foods and avoid dairy products, fatty foods and oils. Don't drink cold or icy drinks, but choose hot and warm ones instead.

This is the season when everyone is likely to feel sluggish, dull and heavy. Regular morning exercise is most important. Saunas are also beneficial at this time of year. Towards the end of the season, in the spring, is one of the best times to take the three-day detoxifying program (see pages 70–3) or take a course of panchakarma at an ayurvedic spa (see page 130). This is the time of year when mental stimulation is most needed, too, so seek out interesting company and activities.

Changing seasons

While each of the doshic seasons has particular qualities and its weather conditions affect us in different ways, perhaps the most disruptive times in the year are those when one season changes to the next. The effects can be physical, mental and emotional. If, for instance, you are pitta/vata, the change of season from summer to autumn is a particularly vulnerable time. During this two- to three-week period, you should not start up any new ventures or put yourself under pressure. It is especially important at this time to keep to a good diet and to a daily routine and, if at all possible, to take a relaxing break or vacation.

However, while there are periods that you are more vulnerable than others, by keeping in balance you can minimize any troublesome effects. These seasonal changes are simply times of transition and, as long as you swim with the tide, rather than battling against it, they shouldn't cause you any problems.

The cycle of life

The doshas also work in a larger time-frame than through days and seasons, with particular doshas playing more significant parts in different stages of our lives. Childhood and early adulthood are our kapha period. Kapha builds our bones and muscles as we grow, until we reach the peak of our physical strength. Pitta gives us the focus and ambition we need in order to achieve our adult goals. Vata governs the third stage of our lives, reducing the need for sleep as we get older and granting us insight and perception.

The qualities and the potential illnesses of each dosha can be observed in these three key stages of life. During childhood, we need more sleep and constant nourishment to grow strong bones and healthy tissues. Childhood is also often punctuated by colds and sinus problems: ear infections, asthma and other typical forms of kapha congestion. The pitta adult period is the time when we are most driven. It is also, therefore, the time when stress-related illness is most likely: heart attacks, ulcers and high blood pressure, as well as digestive acidity. During the vata adult period, our bodies become drier and often lighter. Many people observe that their skin becomes very dry, but this vata effect happens

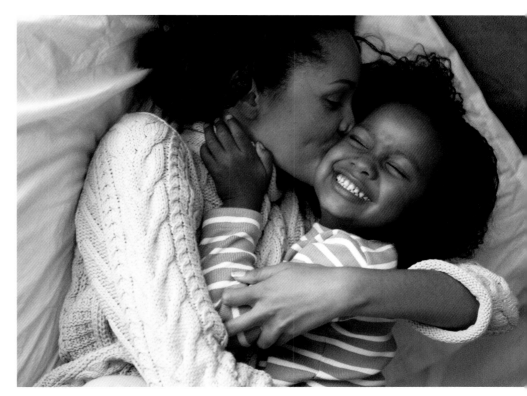

Childhood and early adolescence are our kapha period.

internally, too, so that extra lubrication – particularly of the joints – is needed. You can supply this with gentle exercise, especially yoga, and a daily self-massage with sesame oil (see pages 134–7). Of course, when you take steps to counter these tendencies of the seasons of the year and of your own life, you can balance out the risks of all these ill-effects.

PART TWO

Your
home spa

Now that you have worked out your unique combination of doshas, together with any doshic imbalances you may have, you are ready to set out on the path to health and harmony. To create this state of health and happiness, you need to try to put your life in balance in several key areas. European ayurveda does not work on quick-fix principles. Think of it not so much as a visit to a health spa during which you feel cleansed and relaxed for a few days—only to return to all your worst habits as soon as you get home! Instead, you are going to a spa for life, one that is tailored to your unique needs and environment. Your home spa involves the three key areas that were featured in the questionnaire: your diet, your body and metabolism, and your mind and emotions.

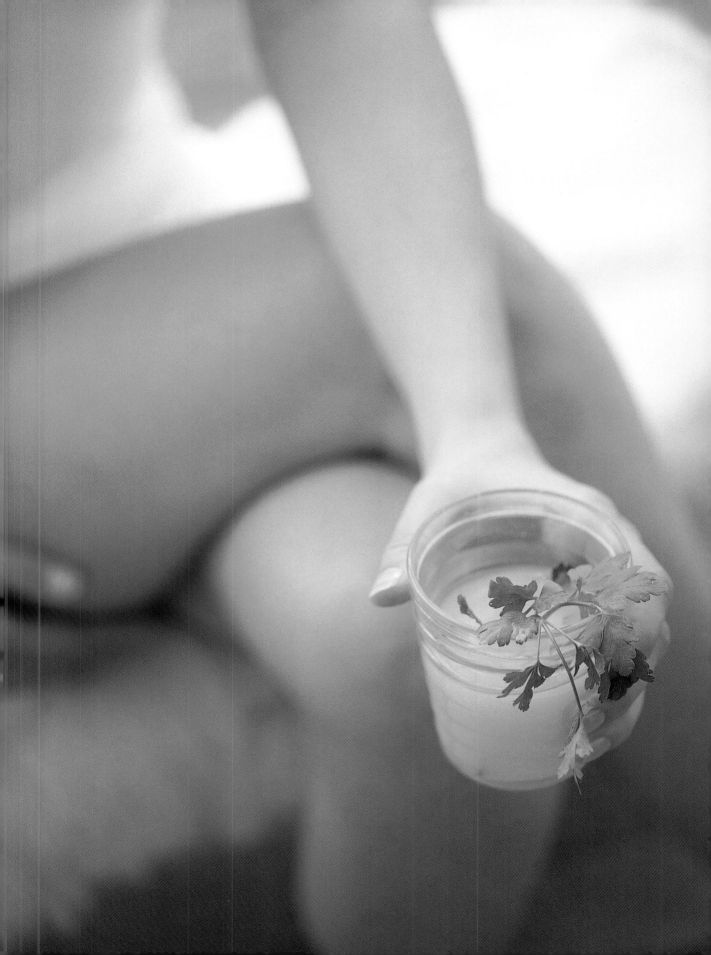

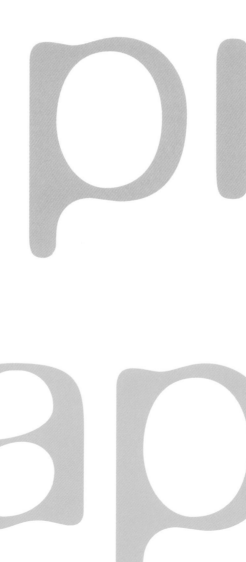

Chapter four

The food spa

In ayurveda, food *is* medicine and its impact on your health cannot be over-emphasized. It is nowadays generally recognized by Western medical practitioners that particular foods— taken in excess or missed out from the diet altogether—can lead to particular diseases. For instance, the risks of stroke and heart attack are known to be increased by a diet that is too high in fat, while the World Health Organization has linked a lack of fruit and vegetables with certain types of cancer.

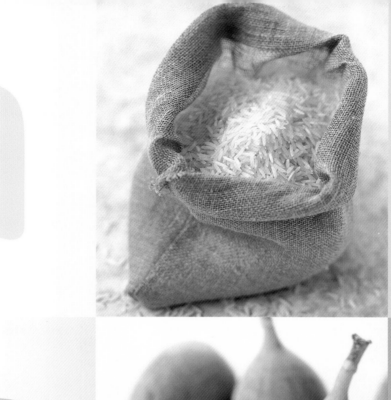

Vata food

Qualities to favor:
warm, oily, heavy, sweet, sour, salty

Qualities to reduce:
cold, dry, light. bitter, astringent

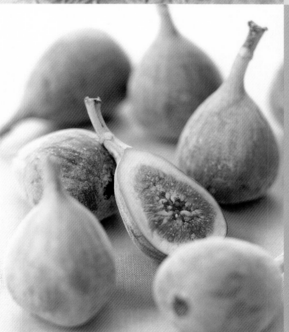

Pitta food

Qualities to favor:
sweet, bitter, cool, astringent, heavy

Qualities to reduce:
pungent, salty, sour, light, excessively oily—above all, Pittas should avoid acidic foods

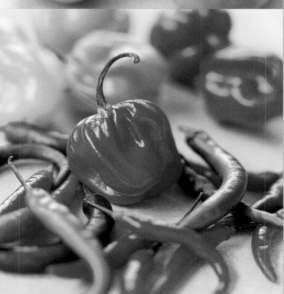

Kapha food

Qualities to favor:
light, dry, warm, spicy, bitter, astringent

Qualities to reduce:
heavy, oily, cold, sweet, salty, sour

Food as medicine

In ayurveda the principle of food as medicine is not based simply on the nutritional qualities of certain foods. The whole food—not just particular constituents of it—is regarded as having a beneficial or harmful effect on the individual.

The emphasis here is on the individual, as certain foods can be good or bad for you, depending on your doshic makeup. So one person's meat really can be another's poison. You will find the general guidelines for pacifying doshic dietary imbalances on pages 56–61.

However, you should bear in mind that these are just guidelines. As you become more attuned to how your body reacts to food on a day-to-day basis, you may notice more subtle responses in yourself—and it is these you should listen to above all else.

Ama and agni

Good food and digestion are of central importance in ayurveda because the end-product of poorly digested food, known as ama, is regarded as one of the main culprits in causing disease. Ama is often translated into English as "toxins" but it is, in fact, more far-reaching than this, although toxins are certainly part of ama. Because ama clogs up the system, it makes all the bodily processes sluggish and less efficient—leading, in turn, to a further build-up of ama.

When food is properly digested and metabolized, there is less risk of ama, so good digestion is very important in ayurvedic thinking. The body's ability to digest and metabolize is governed by agni, the digestive force or fire that can convert food to energy. Different people will have a weak or strong agni, making them less or more able to digest their food well. The Pitta agni is usually the strongest, while Vata has a more unpredictable digestive fire and Kapha has the slowest.

Food should be delicious

Food should, quite simply, be delicious, with a combination of smells and tastes that is irresistibly tempting! Just as animals in the wild seek out foods with particular medicinal properties by their taste and smell, human beings, too, can learn to balance their diets by balancing a variety of tastes. These should, of course, be the real tastes of the whole foods, not those of artificial additives designed to tempt jaded palates.

Ayurveda recognizes six different taste groups (see pages 54–5) and, if a meal lacks one or more of the tastes, it will ultimately be unsatisfying and you will crave the missing taste. Hence the dilemma of the dieter who eschews sweet foods at meal-times in an attempt to lose weight and ends up bingeing on chocolate later.

In general, European ayurveda favors organic foods that have not been subjected to chemical contamination and a preponderance of cooked foods rather than raw ones because they tend to be easier to digest.

Eating with attitude

It is not only what you eat that is significant. Just as vital is how and when you take your meals. The main meal of the day should be lunch, while both breakfast and supper should be light as you will be eating them during kapha time, when your digestion is at its weakest.

Always focus on your food at mealtimes—don't be distracted by reading or watching television. Eat slowly, chewing your food thoroughly, and take time to savor and enjoy the tastes. Pitta types find this quite difficult as they have a tendency to eat too quickly, with resulting indigestion. Make a conscious effort to put down your fork between mouthfuls and not to pick it up again until you have swallowed. Gulping down food also means gulping down air, so that excess vata gets into the digestive system, causing wind and bloating. Don't overeat. You should be three-quarters full at the end of a meal, and five hours to complete. If you feel hungry, have something very light, such as fruit or fruit juice. Alternatively, a teaspoon of honey in warm water will restore your energy and pacify hunger pangs.

Finally, ayurveda advises warm or room-temperature food and drink. Cold and iced drinks damp down the digestive fire needed for proper metabolism of food.

It is better to eat the **wrong food** with the **right attitude,** than the right food with the wrong attitude.

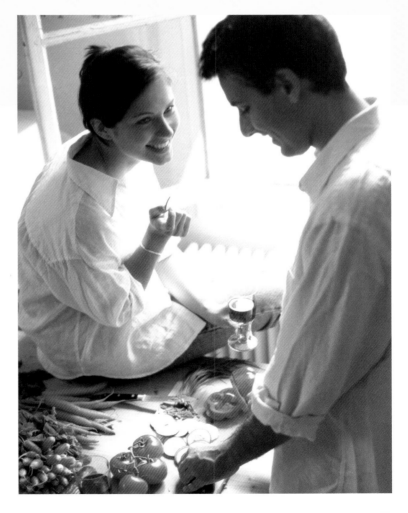

but you won't be able to judge this properly if you eat too quickly. At the end of a meal, sit quietly for a few minutes and then take a short walk (five to ten minutes) to aid digestion and calm the mind.

Your emotions affect your digestion too. You should always try to eat in a comfortable, quiet environment, and put off eating if you are angry or upset—such feelings can sour the food in your stomach. According to ayurveda, the person preparing the food should also feel tranquil and unhurried during the cooking process for it to have the maximum benefit.

Snacks between meals will disrupt the digestive process, which normally takes between three

The ayurvedic taste groups

According to ayurveda, every food belongs to a particular taste group and, for a balanced, healthy diet, you need to have something from each group at every meal.

This variety of tastes ensures both stimulation of the digestive system and better digestive absorption. A diet that concentrates on one particular kind of food will not be properly balanced and can lead to a whole host of ailments. An obvious, all too common example of this problem is the high salt and fat content of the processed foods that are so popular in the West today and that bring with them obesity, high blood pressure and heart disease.

Ayurveda divides food into six groups – sweet, sour, salty, pungent, bitter and astringent. The way individual foods are categorized may seem strange at first. Most people would probably not regard milk or bread as sweet, for instance. However, the groupings are governed not just by taste but by the ultimate effect of a particular food on the physiology and, as with all aspects of ayurveda, balance is the key.

Pacifying imbalances

Food is a therapy in itself. This includes not just the types of food that we eat, but the way in which we eat them and how we stimulate our digestive systems for optimum absorption of the nutrients. You should always follow the diet plan that relates to your principal dosha—as indicated by your answers to the A questions in the Digestion section of the questionnaire. Your answers to the B questions, if they indicate a different dosha than the As, tell you your imbalance. In this case, continue to follow the diet plan for your principal dosha, but incorporate the following advice into *how* you eat and drink.

the six groups

6

SWEET
- *milk, cream, butter, ghee*
- *sweet fruits (mangoes, dates, figs, etc.)*
- *cooked root vegetables*
- *dried beans and lentils*
- *bread and grains*
- *sugar*

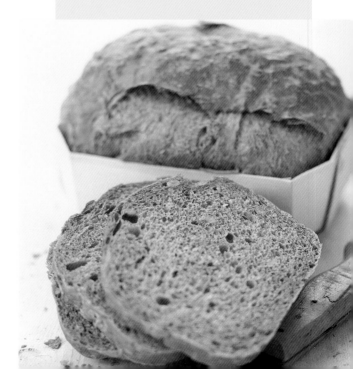

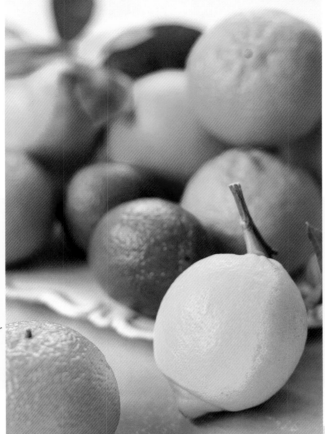

SALTY
- *salt*
- *snack foods (chips, etc.)*

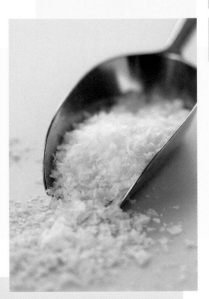

SOUR
- *citrus fruits*
- *fermented milk products (yoghurt, cheese, etc.)*
- *wine, vinegar*

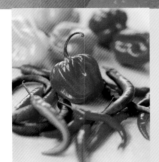

PUNGENT
- *hot-tasting vegetables, such as onion and radish*
- *hot-tasting spices and flavorings (garlic, chilli, pepper)*

BITTER
- *olives*
- *cooked, green, leafy vegetables*

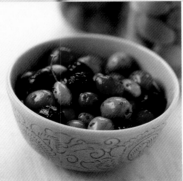

ASTRINGENT
- *nuts*
- *honey*
- *raw vegetables*
- *unripe fruits, apples, berries*

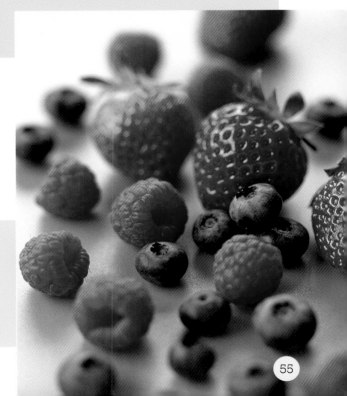

Pacifying a **vata** imbalance

Vatas often have an unpredictable or weak digestion and suffer from gas and bloating. For this reason, beans and pulses are not recommended for anyone with excess vata. As part of establishing a routine as well as maintaining energy levels, mealtimes should be as regular as possible, with the main meal at mid-day when pitta—and hence digestion—are at their strongest. For breakfast, have porridge, stewed fruit, toast with ghee and jam, a morning energy drink (see page 63) and herbal tea or hot water. Tea and coffee should be avoided. Vatas should eat organic, unprocessed, vata-pacifying foods. In general, the rule of thumb for Vatas is to favor food and flavors that have qualities opposite to those of vata and to eat larger quantities of food than you usually do. This will bring the vata digestion into balance.

Qualities to **favor**
- Warm, oily, heavy, sweet, sour, salty

Qualities to **reduce**
- Cold, dry, light, bitter, astringent

Keeping it in proportion

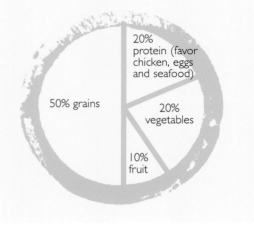

- 20% protein (favor chicken, eggs and seafood)
- 50% grains
- 20% vegetables
- 10% fruit

Tips for pacifying **vata**

- Take ginger pickle fifteen to twenty minutes before all your meals to stimulate the digestive juices.
- Eat regular meals.
- Do not snack between meals.
- Before eating, relax for five to ten minutes.
- Focus all your attention on your food while eating —don't read, work or watch TV at the same time.
- Eat in a quiet, peaceful atmosphere.
- Drink only hot or warm food and drink— nothing cold or with ice.
- Avoid stimulants such as coffee and fizzy drinks.

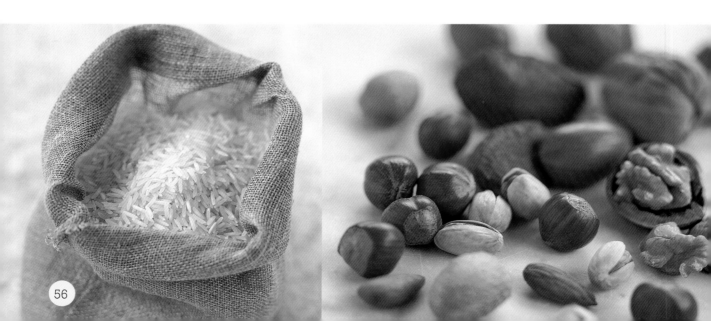

Vata-pacifying foods

Dairy	All dairy products help to reduce excessive vata. Drink milk warmed and only with other sweet foods, not with a meal that comprises a variety of tastes.
Grains	Favor basmati rice, wheat, cooked oats. Reduce barley, corn, millet, raw oats (in muesli) and rye.
Sweeteners	Honey, raw sugar, molasses, brown sugar, maple syrup.
Vegetables	Favor cooked rather than raw vegetables. Beets, carrots, sweet potatoes, garlic, green beans and pumpkin are good for Vatas. Small amounts of green leafy vegetables, celery and potatoes can be eaten, but sprouts and salads are unsuitable.
Fruit	Sweet, sour, heavy fruits are good, especially bananas, avocados, peaches, cherries, mangoes, pawpaws and figs. However, dry, light and astringent fruits should be reduced, in particular apples, pears, cranberries and dried fruits.
Beans	Vata types should avoid dried beans, though lentils, mung beans and tofu can be eaten in moderation.
Nuts	Vatas can eat all nuts in moderation.
Meat & fish	Chicken, seafood and turkey are good for Vatas, but you should avoid red meat.
Oils	All oils are good for Vatas.
Herbs & spices	All spices are good for Vatas, particularly cinnamon, coriander, cardamom, cumin, saffron, salt and fresh ginger.

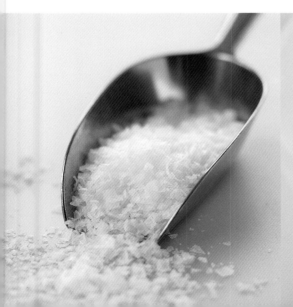

Pacifying a pitta imbalance

The Pitta type has a digestion that is both strong and regular. It is important for Pittas to have a satisfying meal at midday, when pitta is at its strongest, otherwise your stomach will become too acid and this will cause considerable discomfort. Breakfast is important, too, and Pittas should never be tempted to skip it. Choose cereals with milk, porridge, stewed fruit, toast with ghee and jam—but never have a fried breakfast or coffee or regular tea. Peppermint tea is very cooling for Pittas and should be drunk at breakfast and throughout the day. Pittas should eat organic, unprocessed, pitta-pacifying foods. In general, the rule of thumb for Pittas is to favor food and flavors that have qualities opposite to those of pitta—hot, sharp, bright, liquid, slightly oily and sour. This will bring the pitta digestion into balance.

Qualities to favor
■ Sweet, bitter, astringent, heavy, cool

Qualities to reduce
■ Pungent, salty, sour, light, excessively oily— above all, Pittas should avoid acidic foods

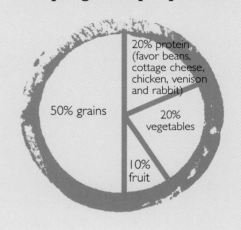

Keeping it in proportion

50% grains

20% protein (favor beans, cottage cheese, chicken, venison and rabbit)

20% vegetables

10% fruit

Tips for pacifying pitta

■ Eat slowly.
■ Do not overeat.
■ Do not snack between meals.
■ Do not miss meals.
■ Do not work, watch TV or read while eating.
■ Always eat sitting down.
■ Eat your main meal at lunchtime.
■ Stay seated and resting for five minutes after finishing a meal.
■ Drink peppermint tea after meals.
■ Avoid alcohol.
■ Eat calmly—if you are feeling angry or upset, take time to calm down before you eat.
■ Avoid coffee and fizzy drinks.

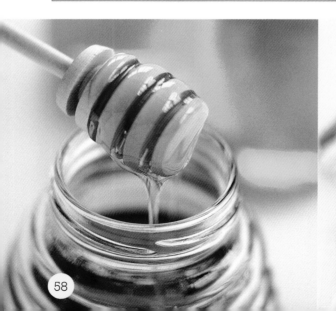

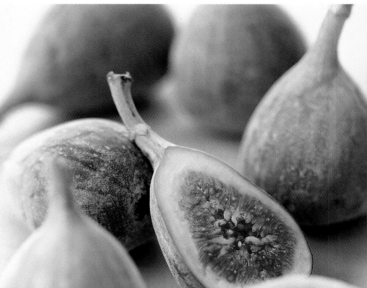

Pitta-pacifying foods

Dairy	Ghee and boiled milk are both very good for Pittas. Sour-tasting foods, such as cheese and yoghurt, should be reduced—in particular, old, hard cheese which will aggravate pitta.
Grains	Favor basmati rice, wheat, oats. Reduce corn, millet and rye.
Sweeteners	Unprocessed sugars are best for Pittas. Maple syrup is excellent and honey in small doses is good too. Palm sugar, also known as jaggery, is very good.
Vegetables	Most vegetables are good for Pittas, with the exception of onions, garlic, hot peppers and tomatoes.
Fruit	All sweet fruit is good, especially grapes and raisins. However, sour, unripe fruits should be reduced, while citrus fruit (except lemons) should be avoided altogether.
Beans	Red lentils can be eaten in moderation by Pittas, but kidney beans and tofu should be avoided.
Nuts	All nuts, except for peanuts, are fine if eaten in moderation.
Meat & fish	Chicken and turkey are good for Pittas, but you should avoid oily fish and red meat.
Oils	Ghee is best—it will actually have a detoxifying effect—and coconut is also good. Moderate amounts of butter and olive oil are fine.
Herbs & spices	Pittas should favor fennel, cinnamon, turmeric, coriander, cardamom, cumin, saffron and fresh ginger. Nutmeg is good too.

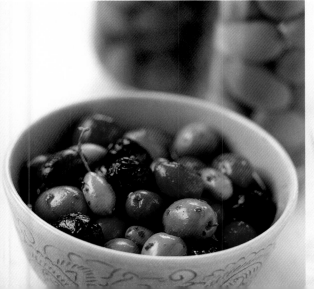
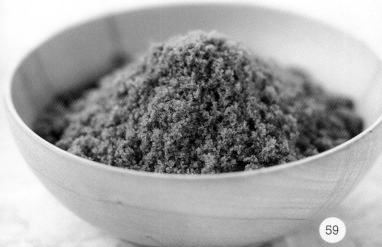

Keeping it in proportion

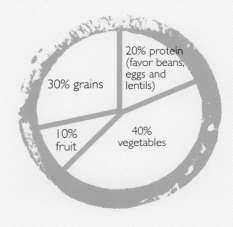

- 20% protein (favor beans, eggs and lentils)
- 30% grains
- 10% fruit
- 40% vegetables

Pacifying a kapha imbalance

Kapha people often have a sluggish digestion and a tendency to overeat, particularly craving sweet and fatty foods. They are the most likely to put on excess weight and they find it hardest to shed it again. Eating late at night will increase the likelihood of weight gain and the main meal should be eaten at midday. Kaphas can skip breakfast if they don't feel hungry and they can also have coffee in the mornings— this is the only dosha to benefit from the stimulation. Otherwise, toast with a little ghee and honey, rice cakes and stewed fruit make a good breakfast, drunk with a warming, stimulating herbal tea with cloves, cinnamon and ginger. Kaphas should eat organic, unprocessed, kapha-pacifying foods, avoiding dairy products because it can lead to excessive production of mucus. In general, the rule of thumb for Kaphas is to favor food and flavors that have qualities opposite to those of kapha.

Tips for pacifying kapha

- Get up early and exercise vigorously to stimulate digestion for the rest of the day.
- If you don't feel hungry, miss breakfast.
- Take ginger pickle before all meals.
- Drink fresh ground coffee in the morning to stimulate the system.
- Avoid all dairy foods and cold fizzy drinks.
- Reduce intake of red meat and all oil.
- Eat your main meal at lunchtime.
- Take a five- to ten-minute walk after eating.
- Do not eat after 7 P.M.

Qualities to favor
- Light, dry, warm, spicy, bitter, astringent

Qualities to reduce
- Heavy, oily, cold, sweet, salty, sour

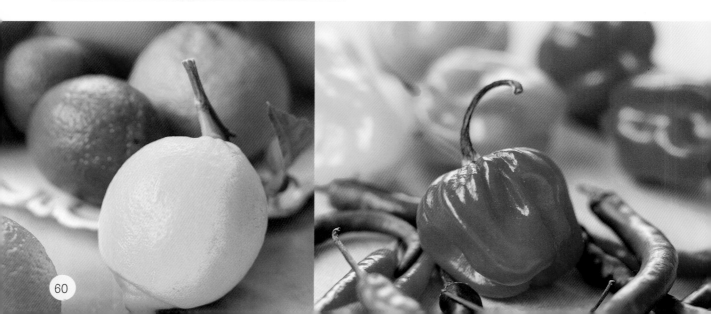

Kapha-pacifying foods

Dairy	Intake of all dairy foods, particularly milk, cheese and butter, should be reduced. Drink low-fat warmed milk only occasionally and never if you have any form of cold or congestion. Do not eat ice cream.
Grains	Grains are good for Kaphas, especially barley, corn and rye, but reduce oats, rice and wheat.
Sweeteners	Kaphas crave sweet tastes but, with the exception of honey, which is astringent, they all increase kapha and should be avoided.
Vegetables	Pungent and bitter vegetables are good for Kaphas, especially broccoli, Brussels sprouts, cabbage, celery, fennel, lettuce, leeks, mushrooms and onions. You should avoid sweet vegetables such as tomatoes, sweet potatoes and zucchini.
Fruit	Light astringent fruits are best—apples, pears, cherries and berries. Avoid sweet, heavy fruits, such as avocados, bananas, figs, dates, coconuts, and all citrus fruits.
Beans	All beans are good, except for kidney beans.
Nuts	Avoid all nuts.
Meat & fish	Meat and fish should be taken very sparingly by Kaphas, eating only the white meat from chicken and turkey and non-oily fish.
Oils	Very moderate amounts of almond and sesame oils are OK, but avoid all other oils.
Herbs & spices	All spices are beneficial for Kaphas, but salt should be avoided.

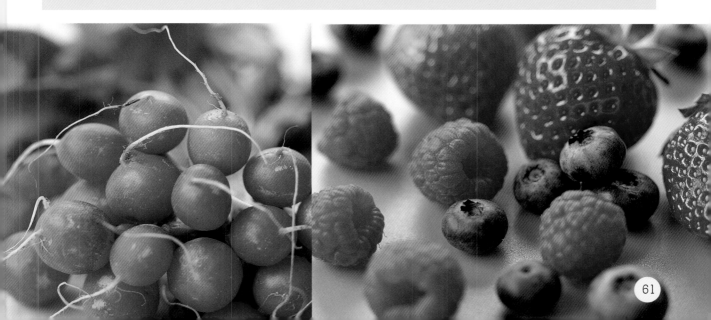

Natural elixirs

There are a number of natural elixirs for promoting health and digestion, boosting energy and calming the mind. The ones on these pages are easy to prepare and to incorporate into your daily spa routine, and you should notice a definite improvement if you take them on a regular basis.

Ginger pickle

Eating ginger pickle half an hour before meals stimulates and balances the digestive system. This helps you extract maximum nutrition from the food and reduces the chances of undigested food (ama) building up in the system. Vatas should take it before both lunch and dinner, while Kaphas should take it in the morning too. Pittas also benefit from ginger pickle, unless there is a severe excess of pitta in the system or in cases of stomach upset and diarrhea.

For one day
2 tsp fresh lemon juice
2 tsp honey
pinch salt
2 heaped tsp grated fresh ginger

1 Add the lemon juice, honey and salt to the ginger.
2 Mix together well.
3 Take 1 tsp of the pickle as a digestive aid twenty to thirty minutes before lunch and the evening meal.

For one week
Half a 1lb (454g) jam jar of fresh ginger
Lemon juice to cover the ginger
Honey as required
Salt as required

Mix all the ingredients together as above. Store in a refrigerator and stir before taking, as before.

Bedtime drink

This is a very settling drink to ensure a good night's sleep. It is particularly recommended for Vatas and Pittas but is also suitable for Kaphas if it is not kapha season and if you do not suffer from sinus problems or have a cold, congestion or excess mucus.

⅔ C (150ml) milk or milk and water
2 heaped tsp fresh grated ginger

8–10 raisins
½–1 tsp ghee
1½ inch (1cm) of vanilla pod
Pinch of cardamom
Pinch of turmeric
Pinch of nutmeg

1 Put all the ingredients into a saucepan and slowly bring to a boil.
2 Simmer for 2 minutes.
3 Pour into a cup and drink before going to bed.

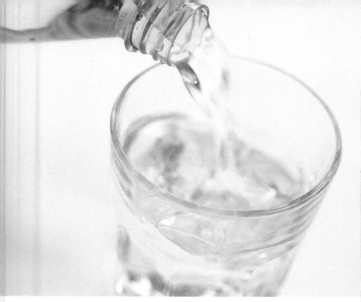

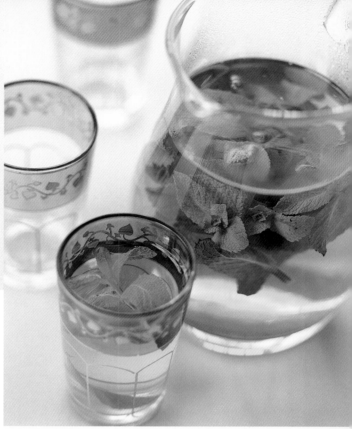

Morning energy drink

Ayurveda regards cows' milk as a very nourishing food, excellent for physical strength, longevity and settling the mind. Boiled and spiced, it becomes more digestible, often overcoming the problems otherwise encountered. This is a good drink for Vatas and Pittas at breakfast-time and is also suitable for Kaphas when it is not the kapha season or weather (winter or cold damp weather). Traditionally in ayurveda, dairy is avoided on the day of the new moon, which increases kapha and therefore also the tendency to put on weight. Consequently, the day of the new moon is a particularly good time for a fluid-only detox day (see page 66).

> ⅔ C (150ml) milk or milk and water
> 2 heaped tsp fresh grated ginger
> 2 fresh dates
> ½–1 tsp ghee
> Pinch of cardamom
> Pinch of turmeric
> Sugar to taste (optional)

1 Put all the ingredients into a saucepan and bring slowly to a boil.
2 Simmer for 2 minutes.
3 Pour into a cup and drink.

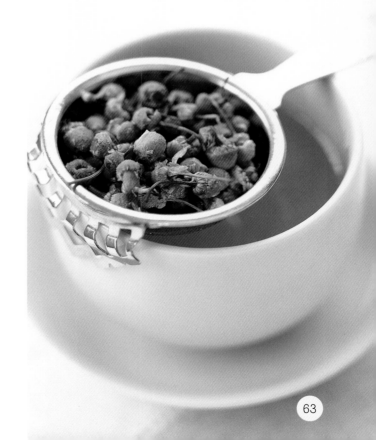

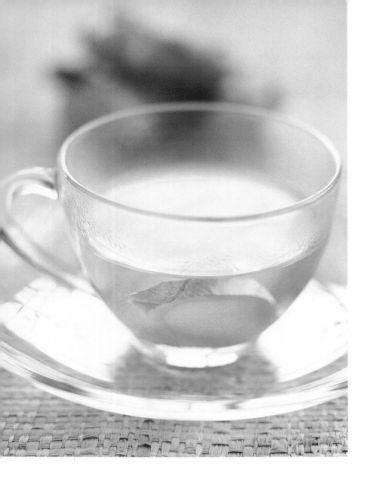

Hot water

Drinking hot water throughout the day helps the body to flush out waste products and prevents dehydration. The water is hot to speed up all the processes involved, in much the same way as washing up in hot water is more effective than in cold. Ideally, boil the water for at least two minutes (it is believed that this puts prana, or life energy, into the water). Drink a minimum of 4 cups a day, sipped regularly every half an hour. Avoid drinking too much within the hour prior to eating a meal, although a teacup during a meal will aid digestion. To vary the taste, Pittas should drink peppermint tea to cool down the system, while Vatas benefit from a slice of fresh ginger in the water.

Churnas

These are doshic seasonings used to flavor your food.
Use the churna appropriate for pacifying your imbalance.

Vata churna

1 heaped tsp cumin
1 level tsp ginger
1 level tsp fenugreek
1 level tsp sugar
½ level tsp turmeric
Pinch of salt

OR

1 heaped tsp cardamon
1 level tsp cumin
1 level tsp ginger
½ level tsp nutmeg
Pinch of hing (asafoetida)
Pinch of salt

Pitta churna

1 heaped tsp fennel
1 heaped tsp cumin
1 level tsp turmeric
1 level tsp coriander
½ level tsp sugar
½ level tsp cardamon
Pinch of salt

Kapha churna

1 heaped tsp ginger
1 heaped tsp black pepper
1 level tsp powdered clove
1 level tsp sugar
1 level tsp coriander
½ level tsp cinnamon
½ level tsp turmeric

Ghee

Ghee is clarified butter, which, according to ayurveda, is one of the foods most beneficial to health, pacifying for all three doshas. It is very pure in nature, increases agni (the digestive fire) and all the digestive energies and enzymes of the body. Unlike other oils and fats, it does not clog the liver, but strengthens it. It is considered beneficial for the eyes taken internally, while there is also a European ayurveda treatment for the eyes using ghee externally.

1 Put 2 sticks (225g) of unsalted butter into a heavy-bottomed saucepan and bring to a simmer over a gentle heat.
2 Cook very slowly for 45 minutes to 2 hours until the butter has turned a transparent golden color. When there are no bubbles, all the water has evaporated and the ghee is ready.
3 Allow to cool a little, then strain the ghee through a muslin cloth into a jar.
4 Use spread on bread or in cooking.

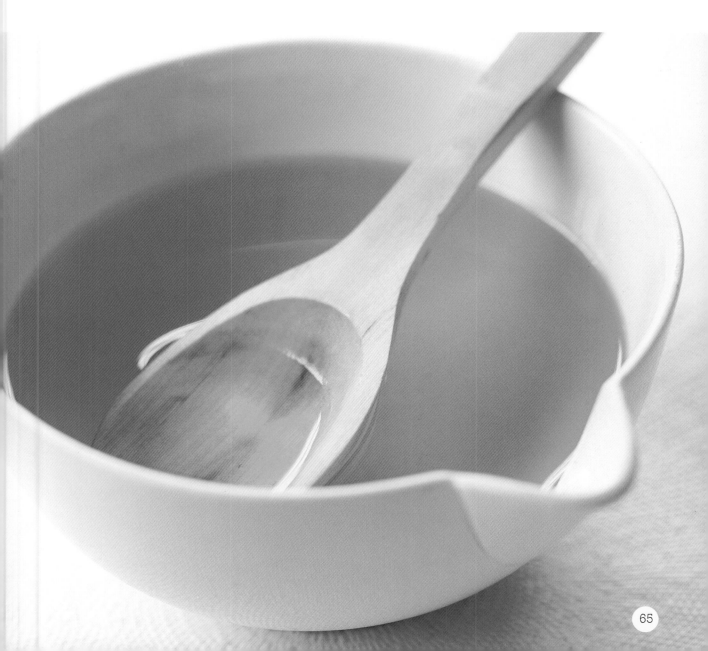

The one-day program

The one-day program is a fluids-only day of cleansing and detoxification. The Peya Soup contains all the proteins and carbohydrates you need for the day. It forms the main part of the diet, flushes toxins out of the system and reduces ama, while balancing and soothing the entire system. The first aim is to cleanse the body, but most people find the program leaves them feeling emotionally and mentally clearer too—producing a real lightness of being. The program should be incorporated into your life on a regular basis. Vatas should have a fluids-only day once every four to six weeks, Pittas every two weeks and Kaphas once a week.

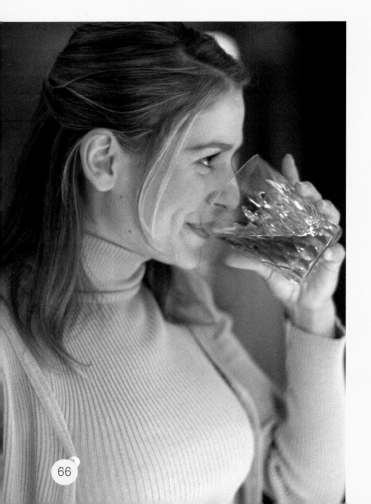

More fluids

During the one-day program, you should have a high fluid intake. Drink a minimum of 4 cups of hot water, preferably more. For added flavoring try fennel tea, ginger tea, cinnamon and cardamon tea. All of these teas are made by infusing the herbs or spices—no black tea is used in them.

Non-acidic fruit juices, such as pear, mango and white grape, are good alternatives, but orange and other citrus juices are too acidic for a detox. Avoid apple juice, too, as this can increase bloating and wind. Drink all juices at room temperature—cold or iced juices will hamper the cleansing process.

If you find soup alone is just not enough, have some toast with a little ghee spread on it. However, try a drink first—thirst is often mistaken for hunger.

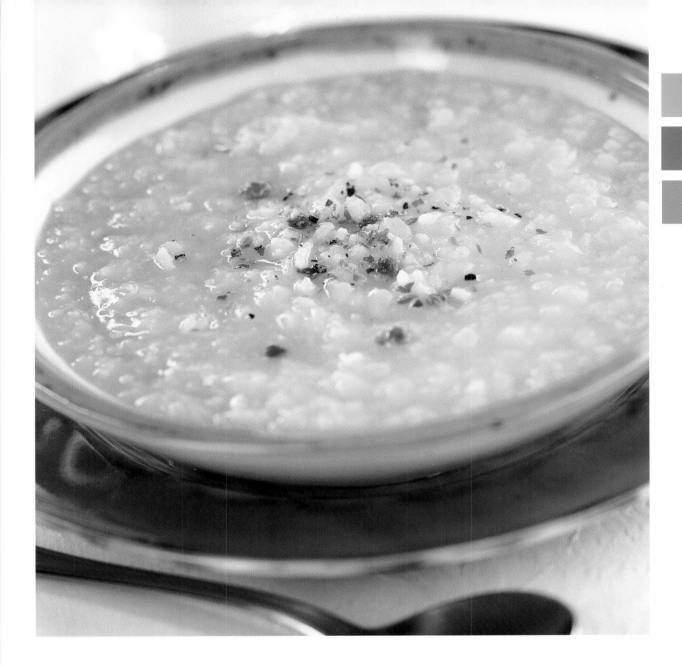

Peya Soup

Serves one

½ C (115g) basmati rice
½ C (115g) yellow mung dhal
2 heaped tsp fresh ginger
½ level tsp turmeric
1 level tsp cumin
Salt and freshly ground black pepper
Tiny pinch of hing (asafoetida)

1 Put the rice and mung dhal into a saucepan and wash well several times.

2 Cover with fresh water and bring to a boil.

3 When the mixture has come to a boil, stir with a whisk until the rice and dhal break down into a smooth consistency. If necessary, add more boiling water until you have a thin soup. Simmer for 20 minutes or until the mixture is completely smooth.

4 Add the other ingredients and cook for a few minutes, stirring the soup well. Serve immediately, or store in a thermos to eat during the course of the day. It can be stored in a flask for 4–5 hours.

Specific recommendations

You are likely to react to the fluid-day differently, according to your dosha. Here are some specific recommendations to make the day as comfortable and beneficial as possible:

Vata

Follow the Daily Routine on pages 108–11 and do not go outside unless it is hot.
■ It is very important for Vatas to stay warm on the fluid day, so make sure your environment is warm and that you eat and drink warm or hot drinks only.
■ If you can spend the day in silence, this is extremely beneficial for Vatas, so turn off the phone or leave your answering machine on.
■ If you find silence difficult, you can play soft music, and artistic or creative activities are recommended, provided that they are not physically demanding.
■ In vata time (2 P.M.–6 P.M.), you would benefit from extra yoga but, if you prefer, simply use the day to rest as much as possible.

Pitta

Follow the Daily Routine on pages 112–15.
■ You need to drink lots of hot peppermint tea during the course of the day—at least 8 cups.
■ If you start to feel unbearably hungry, have some dry toast, but be sure to eat just a little and to eat slowly.
■ Violent films and even the television news should be avoided, but humorous videos are good, as is spending time with friends who lift your spirits and make you laugh.
■ Have a gentle walk in the morning and take the opportunity to pamper yourself—give yourself a manicure or a facial.

Kapha

Follow the Daily Routine on page 116–17.
■ Make sure you get up early and exercise—you have large reserves of energy and exercise won't deplete those even on a fluid day.
■ Drink at least 8 cups of hot stimulating herbal tea, such as ginger and lemon.
■ If you go out, make sure you keep warm and wrap up well.
■ A visit to a steam room is ideal and helps reduce excess kapha.
■ Resist the temptation to sleep during the day, even if you feel tired—do something mentally stimulating instead.

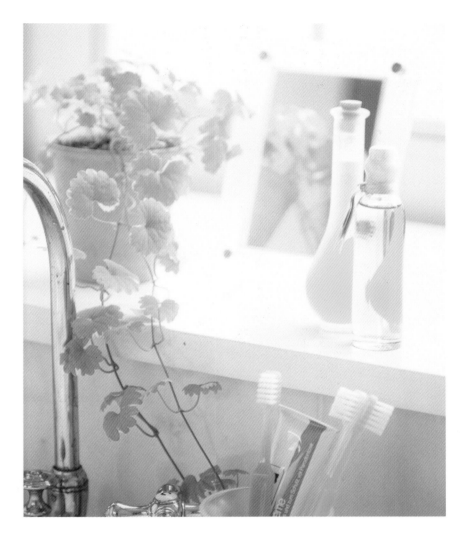

Tongue-scraping

Tongue-scraping dramatically reduces bacteria in the mouth and this in turn reduces gum disease and tooth decay, as well as helping to keep the breath fresh. Brushing the tongue with a toothbrush will disperse the toxins, but it does not remove them from the mouth as effectively as a tongue-scraper. Stainless steel and silver tongue-scrapers are both available (see page 157).

Once you have used tongue-scraping on a one-day program you will see how useful it is to incorporate it into your everyday routine. It is the most effective way of removing that white coat of ama on your tongue in the morning—and that coating is itself a very useful guide to your state of health. If you have a thicker coating than usual in the morning, think back over what you have eaten and at what time you ate it. By a simple process of observation, you will learn what and when foods agree or disagree with you—a perfect self-referral tool. It's also the best restaurant guide you can find! If you have been served processed or reheated food in a restaurant the night before, there will be more ama on your tongue the next morning to prove it.

Using the tongue-scaper

Draw the scraper gently from the back of your tongue toward the tip. Don't start too far back, however, as this can make you gag. Repeat, rinsing the scraper each time for up to thirty seconds.

Day plan

For thousands of years, tongue-scraping has been recommended by ayurveda as an aid to detoxification. Use the technique first thing in the morning, before you clean your teeth, and if you find a white build-up on the tongue (a form of ama) during the day repeat as necessary.

During the course of the day, try to rest as much as you can. It is not a good idea to exert yourself physically or mentally. Meditation and some gentle yoga are both beneficial, but strenuous exercise is not suggested. On fluid days, vata is likely to increase, so take extra care to keep warm and avoid drafty places.

The day following your fluid day, eat a light vegetarian diet.

The three-day program

The three-day program is a comprehensive plan that takes the process of detoxification to a deeper level. It flushes out the system extremely effectively with foods that are light, cleansing and easy to absorb. The profound health-giving effects of ghee are an important part of the plan, but the amount taken depends on your predominant dosha: Kaphas should take the least, Vatas more, Pittas most of all. Ideally, follow the three-day program twice a year for optimum health.

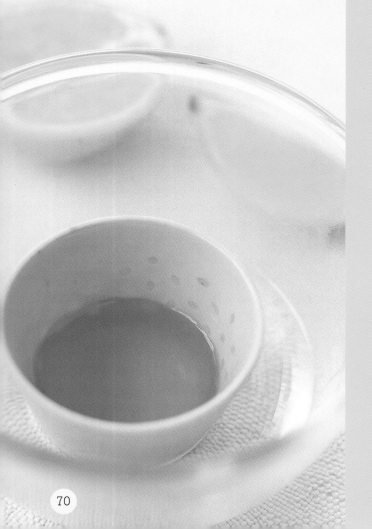

Taking ghee

Ghee subdues your agni (digestive fire), and helps to loosen loosen impurities (ama), moving them out of the deeper tissues into the gastro-intestinal tract by a course of internal oleation.

You can make enough ghee (see page 65) for the whole program in advance and store it in the refrigerator. It will solidify when cool, so you will need to put a cup containing the ghee inside a bowl of warm water until it has melted. While you are waiting, cut an orange or lemon into four sections and fill a thermos with boiling water, adding a 1-inch slice of fresh gingerroot.

When the ghee is a clear golden color it is ready to drink. Gulp it down in one go and then suck on the orange or lemon to take away the taste and oiliness of the ghee. If you do not like the smell, hold your nose as you drink. Afterwards, rest for five to ten minutes and then sip your hot ginger-flavored water—about half a teacup every half-hour—until you start to feel hungry. Don't drink anything for half an hour before eating.

If you find it very difficult taking the ghee in this way, you could try mixing it with half a teacup of milk and a little sugar to taste.

Specific recommendations

Follow the specific recommendations for the one-day program (see page 68), according to your dosha.

Vata
- Start each day with 1 tbsp of ghee on an empty stomach.
- You may feel colder than usual during the program, so stay indoors unless the weather is warm and dry, turn up the heating and wrap up warm.

Pitta
- Start each day with 1½ tbsp of ghee on an empty stomach.
- If this has no effect, increase to 2 tbsp.
- You can talk a gentle walk daily, but don't overdo it and get tired.
- This program clears and cleanses the whole system and you may find that the excess pitta being flushed away makes you irritable, but avoid confrontation at all costs.

Kapha
- Start each day with 1 tbsp of ghee on an empty stomach.
- Exercise daily but don't overdo it and stop if you feel tired.
- As excess kapha is released, you may feel congested and a daily home nasya (sinus treatment, see page 72) will help to relieve this during the course of the program. However, don't repeat the nasya again for at least a week as it is a very powerful process even for a Kapha constitution.
- Don't sleep during the day as this increases kapha.

The best times to undertake the three-day program are during the seasonal changes of winter to spring and summer to autumn. You can extend the detoxification process to a fourth day, following the one-day program (but no ghee on that day).

While on the program, you should go to bed and get up early, and drink a minimum of 8 cups of hot water or the appropriate herbal tea (see page 56–61) each day. Follow your daily routine (see pages 108–17) and also give yourself a sesame oil massage every afternoon between 2 P.M. and 4 P.M. (see page 134), followed by a hot bath. Take time over the massage and be very thorough, massaging every part of your body.

If you are doing the program with a friend or partner, you could give each other a massage. Alternatively, if you are a member of a health club, you could have a massage there, but ask the therapist to use sesame oil and follow the massage with fifteen minutes in the steam room, but not the sauna. Extra meditation is also very beneficial during the program.

Finally, remember that the period immediately after the three-day program is very important too, if you want to gain the maximum benefit. Continue to follow a light diet during the week, with a high fluid intake and plenty of rest. Your appetite will return and you will feel a surge of energy and vitality when the cleansing process is complete.

Home nasya

This is a treatment for anyone who experiences congestion as a result of releasing ama on the three-day program. This is a DIY version of the nasya a therapist would give at a spa, but is still very effective at clearing the sinuses. Excessive mucus can build up to cause pressure headaches, sharp pains behind the eyes and impaired breathing, hearing and sense of taste. Blocked sinuses also result in dullness, heaviness, lack of enthusiasm and even depression.

Mucus is pure kapha and Kapha types are most likely to suffer from it, though a kapha imbalance will produce the same result in the other doshas. If you have this problem, you must keep as warm as possible and the treatment should take place in a warm, draft-free bedroom. Always spit the mucus out into tissues—never swallow it. Avoid dairy, heavy, oily and raw foods for a few days before and a week after nasya. Drinking herbal tea with stimulating flavors will help to expel the mucus, as will a steam room session before and after the treatment.

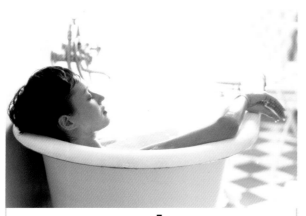

You will need

■ Hot-water bottle ■ Kettle ■ Cup ■ Nasal dropper ■ Olbas oil (from druggist)
■ Nose drops: 1 tsp sesame oil, ¼ level tsp powdered ginger, ¼ level tsp ground black pepper, ¼ level tsp powdered clove, heated slowly in a pan until the powder granules soften. Leave to cool, strain through a muslin cloth and the drops are ready to use.

Nasya procedure

1 Repeat Sun Salutation (see pages 96–103) vigorously for five to ten minutes or until you are sweating freely.

2 With a little warm sesame oil, stimulate the head and neck with a vigorous massage. The faster the movements, the more heat you create —this helps to soften the mucus for expulsion.

3 Put some boiling water into a bowl, add two to three drops of Olbas oil, and sit with your face over the bowl for ten minutes, a bath towel draped over your head to trap the steam. Breathe deeply in and out through your nose and if you can keep your eyes closed, as the steam and Olbas oil may irritate them. Hugging a hot-water bottle to your chest at the same time will also help to remove the mucus. Add more boiling water or Olbas oil, as required, and when you have finished, dry your face thoroughly and quickly so that your face does not get cold.

4 Lie on the bed with your head hanging over the edge, as far back as possible. Place a tissue over your eyes to prevent drops going into them. Using the dropper, put one drop of nasal oil into a nostril, sniffing strongly four or five times. Put five drops into the first nostril, then massage the forehead for one minute. Change to the other side and repeat. If you find the nasal oil is too strong, replace it with plain sesame oil.

5 Repeat steps 3 and 4.

6 Have a hot bath. Just before you get in add five drops of Olbas oil and stay in the bath for ten minutes. Have a box of tissues handy as you may experience a major release of mucus at this point. Dry yourself carefully, keeping as warm as you can, then get into bed with a stimulating hot herbal drink and a hot-water bottle. After nasya you will feel very tired, and you should rest after the treatment and stay indoors for the rest of the day.

Side effects and how to deal with them

The three-day program is a powerfully cleansing and repairing therapy and, while these processes are going on, you may experience certain side effects. These are nothing to worry about—and indeed a good sign that ama is being released—but there are steps you can take to reduce any discomfort.

problem

Headaches
These are usually caused by the elimination of toxins, especially if you have been drinking too much tea, coffee or alcohol before beginning the program. Blocked sinuses, allowing the head to become either too hot or too cold, and too much television, reading or conversation are other possible causes.

General aches and pains
The underlying cause is probably released toxins moving through the body en route to elimination. They can also result from old injuries stored in the body, too much exercise without proper warming up or cooling down, or insufficient rest.

Dull or poor appetite
This is a sign that the body is still focussing on elimination. A heavy diet at this point will slow the process down so keep to a light diet. Rising late or sleeping during the day will increase kapha and dull the appetite. Rest as much as possible.

Lethargy and tiredness
On the program, when you relax deeply, the body has a chance to recuperate, but you may continue to release stored fatigue for some time.

recommendation

- Keep as quiet as possible, avoiding stimulation. Close the eyes and rest for twenty minutes, but don't sleep during the day as this will increase kapha and make the headache worse. If you meditate, ten minutes' practice will help.
- Practice balanced breathing (see pages 126–7) for three to four minutes, or slow, gentle yoga.
- Drink plenty of hot water or herbal tea.
- If it is a sinus or pressure headache, apply Olbas oil to the forehead and temples (but check first that it does not irritate your skin). A steam inhalation is also beneficial.
- If you have tried all of the above without any relief, take aspirin. There is no benefit to be gained from pain.

- Light diet.
- Oil massage.
- Apply a hot-water bottle for ten minutes, then Tiger Balm or Olbas oil to the area of discomfort, followed by a hot bath.
- Keep warm.
- Gentle yoga and Sun Salutation (see pages 96–103), but avoid strenuous exercise.
- Keep fluid intake high (see Headaches for drinks).

- A light diet with well-cooked, easily digested food and ginger pickle is vital to bring back a healthy appetite. Make sure you continue to eat your largest meal at midday and eat very lightly in the evening. Ginger pickle can be taken before all meals until digestion is normal again.
- Avoid raw, cold food and drink. Don't drink anything at all for at least half an hour before meals. At other times, drink hot water flavored with fresh gingerroot.

- Take plenty of rest—early to bed and early to rise.
- Take gentle exercise only.
- Have a light diet, ginger pickle and plenty of hot fluids. A tablespoon of honey in lukewarm water will boost your energy, as will the morning energy drink (see page 63). Avoid stimulating drinks and don't sleep during the day.

Meal plans

Follow the breakfast recommendations for your imbalance (see pages 56–61). Drink a minimum of 4 cups of fluids, during the course of the day, choosing from the same drinks as those on the one-day program. The rest of the recipes for the three days are tri-doshic, or suitable for all types. All recipes are for four people, unless otherwise stated.

day one

LUNCH
Squash burgers
Couscous
Green beans
Mediterranean vegetable slices
Red pepper sauce

Mango and pear fool

SUPPER
Vegetable and barley soup

Pears and golden raisins

SQUASH BURGERS
(makes 8 burgers)
1 C (125g) butternut squash, steamed
¾ C (140g) rice, cooked
1 level tsp sage
Pinch thyme
Salt and pepper
1 heaped tbsp breadcrumbs (made from a thick slice of bread, grated in food processor)
Ghee

1 Briefly mash the first 5 ingredients together. Mold into 8 balls.
2 Roll the balls lightly in the breadcrumbs, to cover, and pat each ball with a palette knife into the required shape.
4 Drizzle with ghee and bake at 400°F (200°C) for 50 minutes, turning them over halfway.

COUSCOUS
1½ C (170g) couscous
1 heaped tsp salt
Juice of 1 lemon
1½ C (350ml) water
1 grated zucchini

1 Mix all the ingredients, put in an oven-proof dish, cover and leave to soak for 30 minutes.
2 Bake in the oven on 325°F (170°C)for 45 minutes. Check and stir several times.

GREEN BEANS
Top and tail 8½oz (250g) of beans and boil in slightly salted water until cooked.

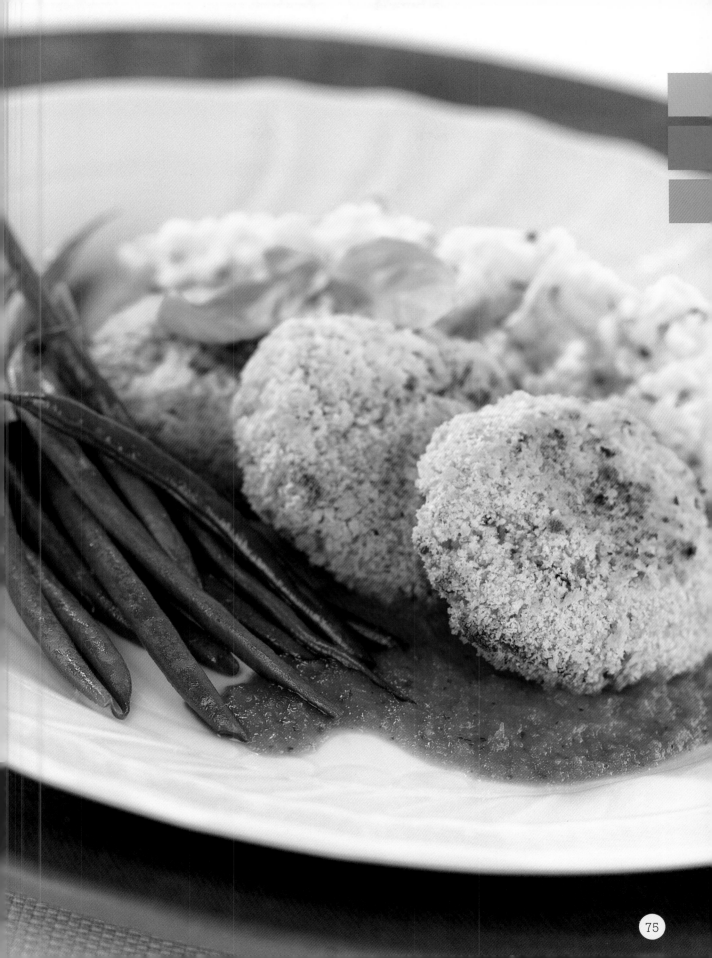

MEDITERRANEAN VEGETABLE SLICES

3 medium zucchini
1 large eggplant
1½ tbsp ghee
1¼ C (300ml) hot water
1 heaped tsp thyme
1 heaped tsp basil
1 level tsp oregano
1 bay leaf
1 heaped tsp salt
1 heaped tsp grated beet
1 heaped tsp turmeric

1 Roughly peel the zucchini and chop them into thick slices.
2 Chop the eggplant into pieces of the same size.
3 Stir-fry them in the ghee on a medium to high heat for 10 minutes, adding splashes of hot water as they become dry.
4 Add the thyme, basil, oregano, bay leaf, salt and water, and simmer for 25 minutes. Cover with a lid and simmer for a further 25 minutes.
5 Add the grated beet and turmeric and shape into slices.
Note: This dish can also be baked in the oven. Mix all of the ingredients, place in a covered oven-proof dish, cover and bake at 350°F (180°C) for 45 minutes.

RED PEPPER SAUCE

½ beet, grated
2 red peppers, roughly diced
1 small zucchini, diced
Juice of 2 carrots
1 heaped tsp thyme
1 heaped tsp oregano
1 level tsp basil
1 heaped tsp salt
Pepper

3¾ C (850ml) water
⅔ C (150ml) soya milk

1 Put all of the ingredients except the soya milk into a saucepan, bring to a boil and simmer for 30 minutes.
2 Blend together in a food processor and add the soya milk. Reheat to serve.

MANGO AND PEAR FOOL

3 mangoes
6 medium pears
1 vanilla bean, chopped
Juice of 3 apples

1 Peel and chop the fruit and place in a saucepan.
2 Add the vanilla bean and apple juice and cook over a low heat for 30 minutes.
3 Put the mixture into the food processor and blend until very smooth.

VEGETABLE AND BARLEY SOUP

⅓ C (75g) pot barley, soaked for at least 2 hours, washed and strained
1 heaped tsp salt
1 heaped tsp freshly grated or finely chopped ginger
9 C (2 liters) water or stock
½ small sweet apple, chopped
1 heaped tsp raisins
1 carrot, peeled and shredded
½ small fennel bulb, finely chopped
6 baby corn, quartered
8 green beans, sliced
1 level tsp cumin
1 heaped tbsp finely chopped fresh oregano
2 heaped tbsp finely chopped fresh parsley
Pinch of hing (asafoetida)

1 Dry-fry the barley with half the salt and the ginger for 1–2 minutes, stirring all the time.
2 Add 2 C (500ml) of water or stock and slowly bring to a boil. Stir the mixture then simmer for 1 hour on a low heat, adding more stock if necessary. Stir occasionally.
3 Meanwhile coat the fruit and vegetables with the herbs and spices and set aside for 10 minutes.
4 Dry-fry the fruit and vegetables and add the barley, which should now be fluffy.
5 Add 1¼ C (400ml) of water or stock, bring to a boil and cook until the liquid has almost disappeared. Then add the rest of the water or stock and cook for 30 minutes over a low heat, stirring from time to time.
6 Liquidize and serve.

PEARS AND GOLDEN RAISINS

½ vanilla bean
4 medium pears, peeled, cored and sliced
20 golden raisins, pre-soaked
1¼ C (300ml) water

1 Split the vanilla bean down the middle with a sharp knife and remove the black seeds. Use both the seeds and the empty bean in cooking.
2 Place all the ingredients in a saucepan and cook very gently for 20 minutes until the pears are sodt all the way through.

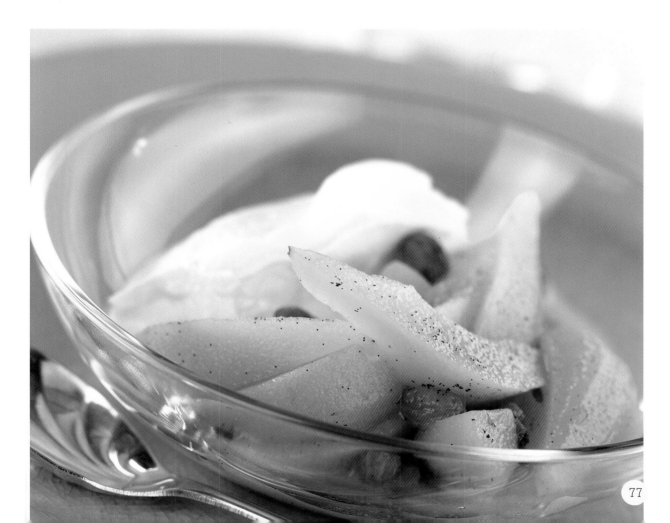

day two

LUNCH
Mediterranean risotto
Broccoli
Beet
Coriander and orange sauce

Apricot purée

SUPPER
Pasta and mixed vegetable soup

Stuffed apples

MEDITERRANEAN RISOTTO
2 cloves
I heaped tsp oregano
2½ tbsp ghee or 2 tsp of olive oil
2 handfuls finely chopped vegetables
(peppers, fennel, celery, carrot, beet,
zucchini, eggplant)
½ C (115g) basmati rice
Handful of raisins
2 bay leaves
I heaped tsp turmeric
I level tsp basil
2 heaped tbsp chopped fresh herbs
I level tsp thyme
I heaped tsp salt
Sprinkle of ground black pepper
12 black olives, pitted
1¼ C (300ml) hot water

I Fry the cloves and oregano for a few seconds in the ghee or oil and add the chopped vegetables. Stir-fry for 10 minutes on a high heat.
2 Add the rice to the vegetables and continue to stir-fry for 10 minutes.

3 Place the rice mixture and all the other ingredients in a saucepan and add 1¼ C (300ml) of boiling water.
4 Bring to a boil, cover with a lid and simmer over a low heat until the rice is light and fluffy.
5 Leave the risotto to stand off the heat for 5 minutes then serve.

BROCCOLI
Chop into florets and cook in boiling water for 6 minutes with a pinch of salt.

BEET
Grate the beet and cook in a saucepan with a little water for 10 minutes. Add some freshly grated ginger and some grated nutmeg. Stir occasionally and add a little salt and pepper to taste.

CORIANDER AND ORANGE SAUCE
¾ C (70g) mung dhal
4½ C (1 liter) water
I heaped tsp salt
I heaped tsp turmeric
Juice of an orange
2 heaped tsp ground coriander seeds

I Bring the mung dhal to a boil in the water, add the salt and turmeric, and cook for 1½–2 hours until the mixture is very smooth, whisking frequently to prevent sticking.
2 About 10 minutes before the end of the cooking time, add the orange juice and the coriander seeds. Stir thoroughly to mix and serve.

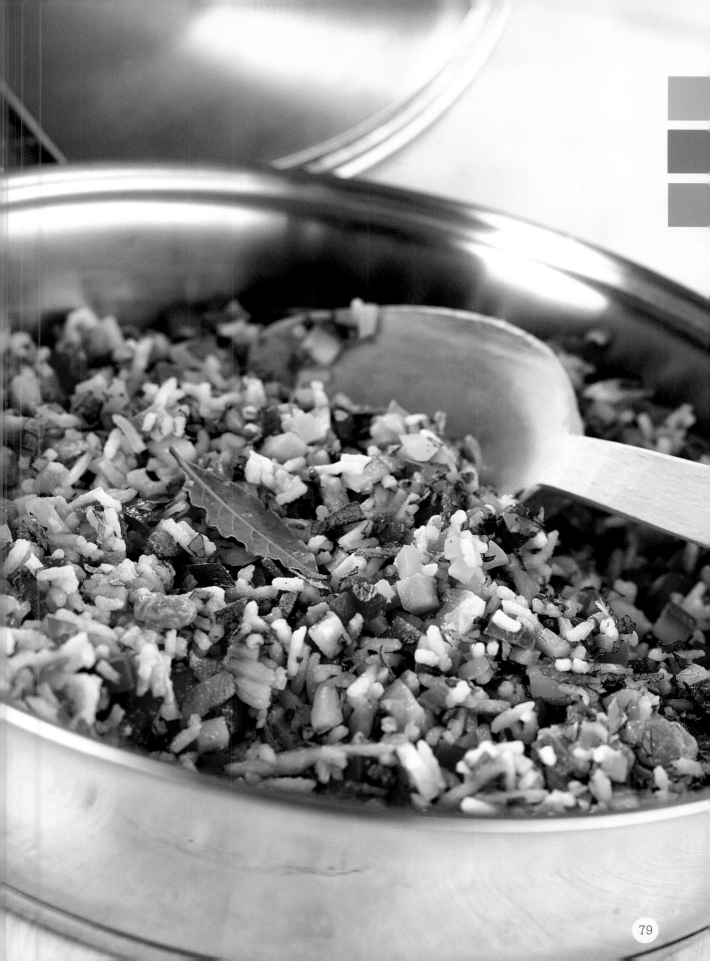

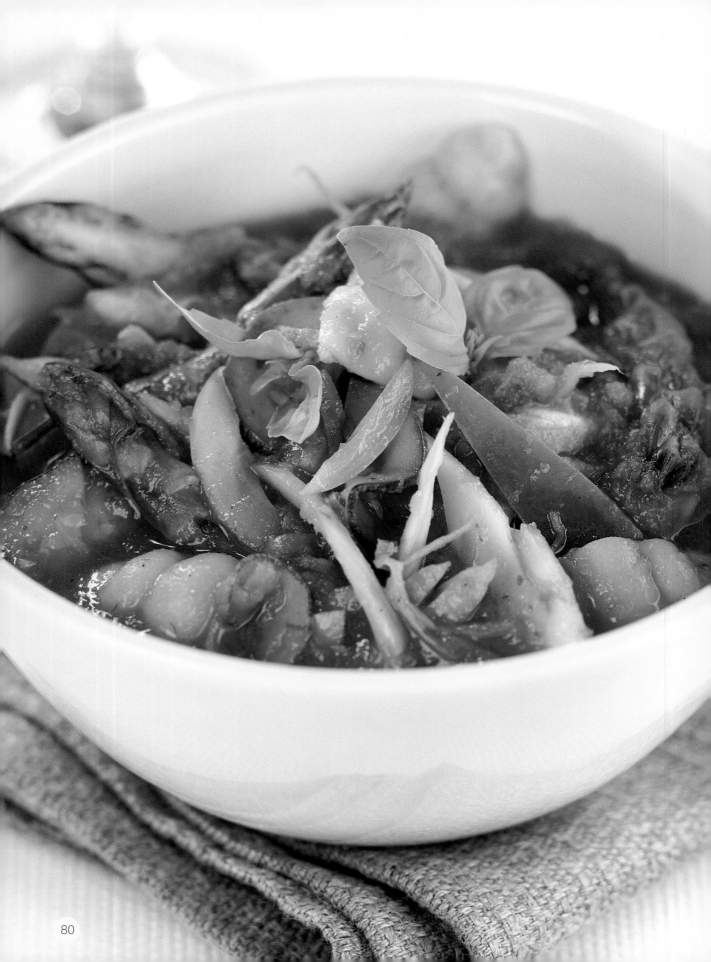

APRICOT PURÉE

2 sweet eating apples, peeled, cored and sliced
½ C (125g) dried apricots, washed and
soaked overnight
½ inch (1cm) vanilla bean
1 tsp rose water
9 C (2 liters) water
4 mint leaves

1 Put all the ingredients except the mint leaves
into a saucepan and bring slowly to a boil.
Simmer, stirring occasionally, for 30 minutes or
until the apricots are soft. The more slowly you
cook them the better, as the flavor intensifies the
longer it takes.
2 Liquidize the mixture, including the vanilla bean.
3 Transfer to small dishes and serve garnished
with a mint leaf.

PASTA AND MIXED VEGETABLE SOUP

9 C (2 liters) stock
2 medium zucchini, peeled and sliced
12 snow peas, halved
2 medium carrots, grated
½ medium fennel bulb, chopped
6 asparagus tips
1 heaped tbsp finely chopped fresh basil
1 level tsp cumin
2½ tbsp Vata Churna (see page 64)
½ level tsp finely chopped fresh mint
¾ C (45g) pasta shells or penne

1 Make the stock and set aside.
2 Coat the vegetables with the herbs and spices
and set aside for 30 minutes.
3 Sauté the vegetables with the herbs and
spices in a large saucepan for 2 minutes, stirring all
the time.

4 Add ⅔ C (150ml) of stock and cook for a further
2 minutes or until the liquid has evaporated.
5 Add the rest of the stock, bring to a boil and
simmer for 45 minutes.
6 Liquidize half of the mixture and return to
the pot.
7 Add the pasta and cook for another 10 minutes
or until the pasta is al dente. Serve.

STUFFED APPLES

4 large apples, such as Golden Delicious
8 dried dates cut into 3 pieces
¼ C (50g) raisins
4 dried apricots
1¼ C (300ml) apple juice

1 Core the apples and make a shallow cut around
the middle of each apple to prevent them exploding
during baking.
2 Fill each apple with dried fruits, place in a small
baking dish and pour around the juice.
3 Cover with foil or a lid and bake at 350°F
(180°C) for 45 minutes. Serve.

day three

LUNCH
Golden pie and herb gravy
Baby corn and green beans

Mixed fruit compote

SUPPER
Spinach soup

Fruit tapioca

3 Barely cover the squash in water and simmer until the water has almost evaporated. Mash thoroughly with a good pinch of nutmeg.
4 Put the vegetables, breadcrumbs and half the lentils on top of the eggplant slices, then spread the mashed squash on top and bake at 375°F (190°C) for 45 minutes.
5 Warm the rest of the lentils in a saucepan with the carrot juice, salt and pepper, cilantro, lemon juice and turmeric. Serve with the pie.

BABY CORN AND GREEN BEANS

Top and tail the beans and the baby corn. Blanch in boiling water for 5 minutes and fry in a little ghee with freshly grated ginger and freshly chopped pineapple. Add salt and freshly ground black pepper to taste.

MIXED FRUIT COMPOTE
4 apples
2 pears
20 dried apricots
2½ C (575ml) apple juice
6 dates
⅓ C (50g) raisins
½ vanilla bean
1 tsp rose water
1 level tsp cinnamon
½ level tsp grated nutmeg
½ level tsp cardamon

1 Peel, core and slice the apples and pears. Place all the ingredients into a pan and bring to a boil.
2 Simmer gently, stirring occasionally, until the apricots and raisins are plump.

GOLDEN PIE AND HERB GRAVY
16 slices of eggplant, ½ inch (1cm) thick and 3 inches (8cm) across
4 good handfuls of finely chopped vegetables: pepper, celery, fennel, carrot, broccoli, zucchini
Ghee
1 heaped tsp thyme
1 heaped tsp oregano
1 heaped tsp basil
2 heaped tsp cumin
2 heaped tsp ginger
1lb (450g) chopped squash flesh
1 level tsp nutmeg
Breadcrumbs made from one slice of bread
1¼ C (225g) cooked red lentils
2 heaped tsp paprika
⅔ C (150ml) carrot juice
Salt and freshly ground black pepper
1 heaped tsp chopped fresh cilantro
Juice of 1 lemon
2 pinches turmeric

1 Steam the eggplant slices until they are just turning soft and place in a single layer on the bottom of a large loaf pan or pie dish.
2 Fry the other vegetables in a little ghee for 15 minutes, adding the herbs, cumin and ginger halfway.

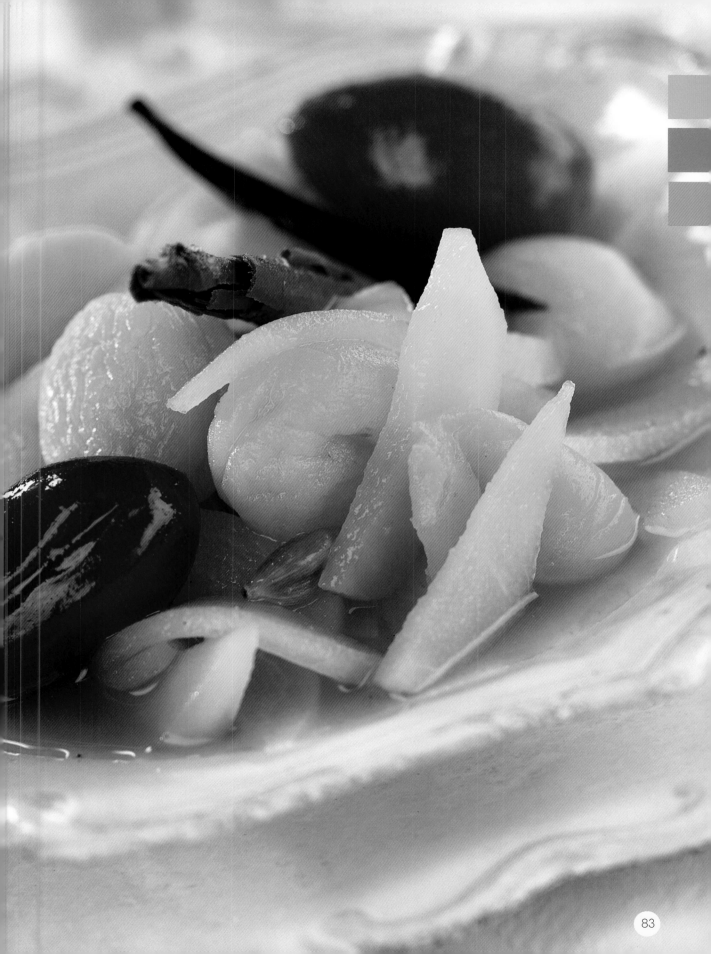

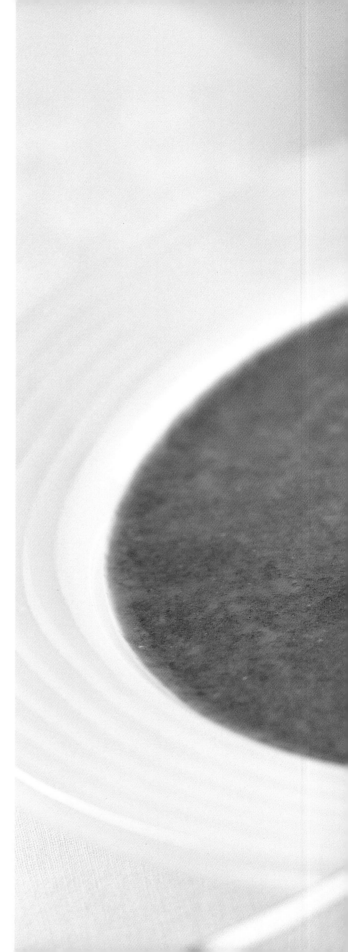

SPINACH SOUP

1½ tbsp ghee
3½lbs (1.5kg) spinach, washed
6 celery stalks, cut into bite-sized pieces
1 C (115g) vegetable bouillon powder
¼ C (50ml) soy sauce
1 heaped tsp unrefined sugar
1 heaped tbsp tarragon
1 heaped tbsp thyme
1 level tsp grated nutmeg
low-fat plain yoghurt

1 Heat the ghee in a large saucepan until it reaches smoking point. Sauté the spinach in the ghee until just tender.
2 Barely cover with water and add all the other ingredients to the saucepan except for the nutmeg and yoghurt. Simmer for about 10 minutes.
3 Remove from the heat and allow to cool slightly. Add most of the nutmeg and blend in a food processor.
4 Serve warm with a sprinkling of nutmeg and a scoop of yoghurt.

FRUIT TAPIOCA

⅓ C (85g) dried apricots, chopped
1⅓ C (55g) small pearl tapioca
1½ C (350ml) fresh organic apple juice
¼ level tsp salt
2½ tbsp maple syrup
1 heaped tsp cinnamon

1 Soak the apricots and the tapioca in the apple juice with the salt for at least 2 hours.
2 Bring to a boil, then reduce the heat and simmer for 5 minutes, stirring constantly.
3 Stir in the maple syrup. Sprinkle on the cinnamon. Cool and serve.

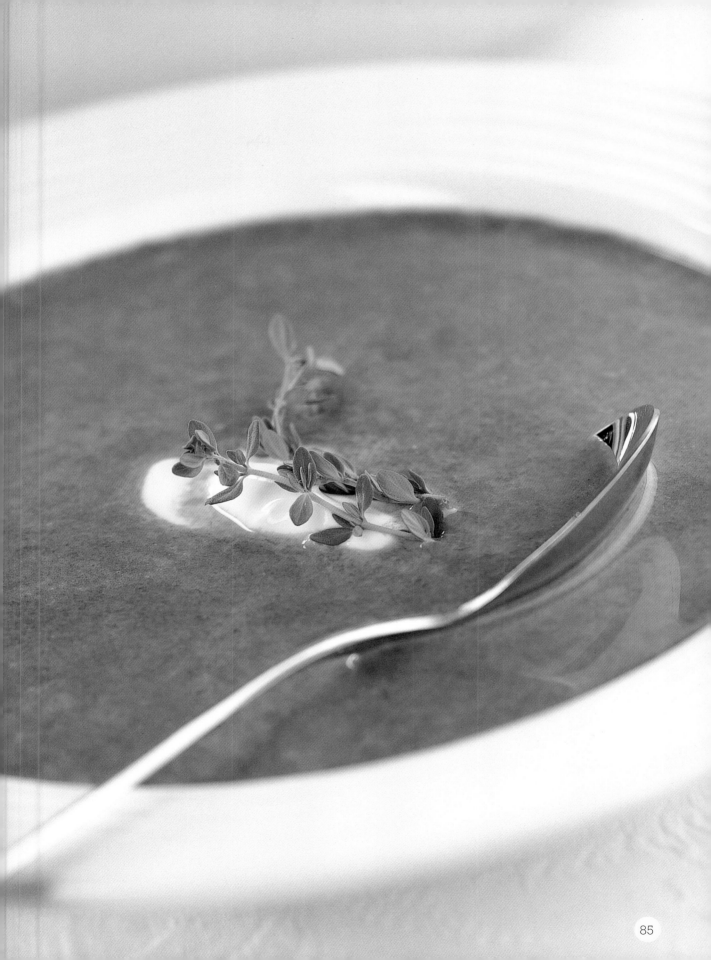

Chapter five

The body spa

Unlike other philosophies of health and fitness, European ayurveda does not take a "one-size-fits-all" approach, aiming to help everyone achieve a similar level of fitness, using the same system and methods for getting there. Instead, it sees each of the doshas as having quite different needs and aims, and suggests radically different solutions for each of them. The one exception to this is yoga, which is beneficial for everyone, although different doshas will take different approaches.

For this section, you should follow the guidelines for your principal dosha, as defined in the Body questionnaire on pages 33–4. If you are mainly Kapha, you need the most vigorous exercise of the doshas. If you are mainly Pitta, you need regular but non-competitive exercise to put you in balance. If you are mainly Vata, you need the most gentle and grounding forms of exercise.

"The body spa" continues to build on the approach of "The food spa" and helps you to work out the best form of exercise for you to feel healthy, fit and balanced. The final part of this chapter gives each dosha its ideal daily routine for maximum health and happiness.

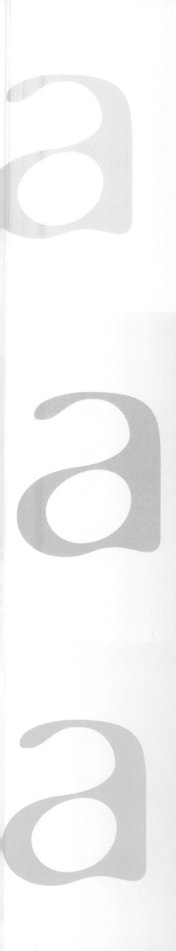

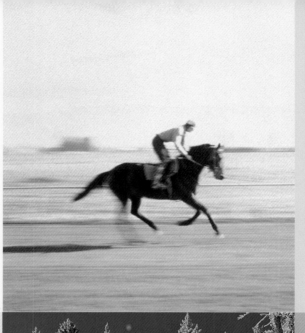

Vata people

Sports:
dancing, gymnastics, badminton, squash, tennis, table tennis, roller-skating, horse-riding, motor-racing

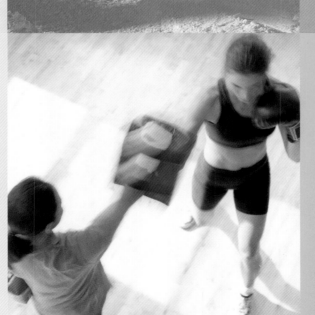

Pitta people

Sports:
golf, sprinting, snooker, archery, skiing, swimming, sailing, windsurfing, paragliding, climbing, yoga, Tai Chi

Kapha people

Sports:
rowing, boxing, wrestling, aerobics, squash, tennis

Your guide to doshic exercise

"No pain, no gain, no brain!"
European ayurveda takes a more gentle view of exercise than is often the case nowadays. Exercising to the point of exhaustion is definitely not to be recommended.

You should always exercise to around 50 percent of your maximum capacity. If you start gasping for air through your mouth, you know you have gone too far. Stop or slow down until you can breathe comfortably through your nose again. You may at first feel that this is slowing you down, but controlling the breath is a crucial element in European ayurveda (this will be discussed in more detail in the next chapter) and correct breathing will ultimately energize and improve your performance, giving you more stamina and a faster recovery time.

Always warm up before you exercise. The Sun Salutation can be used for this as it offers such a comprehensive muscle stretch. It is also just as effective as a final stretch at the end of an exercise session. You can increase the number of repetitions and the speed with which you go through the sequence as you become fitter and looser.

The time of day that you exercise is significant too. You are at the peak of your physical strength between 6 A.M. and 10 A.M., which is kapha time. This is the best time to exercise. From 6 P.M. to around 8 P.M. is also a good time if you cannot exercise during the morning, but exercising after 8 P.M. can disturb your sleep patterns. The worst time to exercise is during the middle of the day from 10 A.M. to 2 P.M. (pitta time) when you are most likely to overstretch yourself, causing potential injuries, and between 2 P.M. and 6 P.M. (vata time), when your body will be at its lowest physical ebb.

vata sports

Vatas do not require strenuous exercise, but should take grounding and calming forms of physical activity instead. Because of your artistic and creative leanings, dancing and gymnastics are very beneficial, as is any gentle exercise performed to music. You do not have a lot of stamina and so marathons, heavy weight-training and vigorous aerobics are inappropriate. However, you do have quick reactions and tend to excel at such sports as badminton, squash, tennis and table tennis. You are also naturally gifted at high jump, long jump, roller-skating, horse-riding and motor-racing. Wind and cold both exacerbate vata, so sailing, skiing and swimming in cold weather should be avoided.

It is particularly important for Vatas not to exercise excessively. Having less stamina than the other doshas, but being naturally enthusiastic, you can easily push yourself too hard without being aware of the fact. This can not only lead you to the point of exhaustion, but also expose you to the risk of injury as you can override your body's warning systems and carry on regardless.

pitta sports

Pittas have moderate physical endurance and, allied with a love of competition, concentration and focus, can excel at sport. In fact, most great sporting champions have a strong will to win, courtesy of pitta. You have a natural ability at all track events, especially sprinting, and excellent hand-to-eye coordination means you are good at golf, snooker and archery. You benefit from activities that cool you down both mentally and physically, so skiing, sailing, swimming and windsurfing are all ideal. The cooling effects of wind and air can be used to advantage with sports such as paragliding, hang-gliding and rock and mountain climbing, where your love of challenge is balanced by being outdoors with panoramic views of natural beauty.

Yoga is a very soothing activity for Pitta types, but you can find it insufficiently challenging sometimes, in which case, Tai Chi and Chi Gung make good substitutes. Highly competitive sports, especially those played indoors, will inflame Pittas, so squash, boxing and kung fu are a nightmare. When pitta is increased by these kinds of sports, Pittas—never the most patient of people at any time—can become irritable and make very bad losers. Once out of balance, Pitta types are determined to win at any cost, and this includes skipping the warm-up and pushing to the point of accident and injury. Generally, Pittas are the most likely dosha to make a good captain.

kapha sports

Kaphas have the greatest reserves of endurance and strength. You are excellent at field sports that require these qualities, such as shot-put, discus and javelin, as well as rowing, boxing, wrestling, weight-lifting and tug-of-war. Aerobics and cardiovascular workouts are particularly beneficial for Kaphas.

Kaphas' biggest battle, though, is to start exercising in the first place. You have a natural urge to take it easy and in cold, wet weather virtually to hibernate. Mental and physical exercise are both vital, however, for Kaphas' well-being and it is more important for Kaphas than the other two doshas to exercise vigorously and regularly. Kaphas are the best team players and you find being in a group stimulating and lifting to your spirits. Being part of a team also helps ensure that you turn up for training sessions! You find solo sports isolating, but playing with a regular partner for squash or tennis is ideal.

The importance of yoga

All three doshas benefit from the regular practice of yoga. It is the perfect way to begin the day, energizing the body and waking up the mind, and once the sequences are learnt and timed to fit your breathing, yoga at its best becomes a form of moving meditation that promotes a feeling of calm and focus.

Over the next eighteen pages, there are different forms of yoga for different standards and abilities. Even if you feel that, due to stiffness, you are not able to do the more usual forms of yoga, you can still do the Yoga in a Chair exercises opposite and benefit from their gentle, rhythmic stretching. If you are able to do Sun Salutation, but you have not exercised for some time, take it very slowly at first, don't over-stretch and try only a couple of repetitions daily until you feel able to do more. As a very rough rule of thumb, Vatas should do five to ten repetitions slowly; Pittas should do the same number, a little more quickly; while Kaphas should do ten or more repetitions as quickly as possible, keeping the breathing rhythmical.

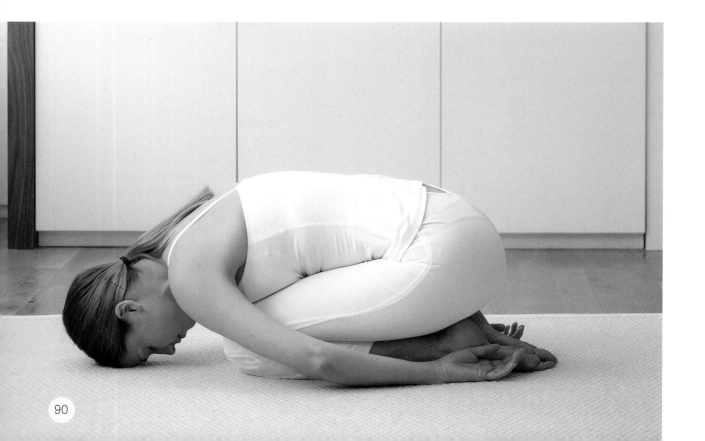

Yoga in a chair

Yoga is accessible to everyone whatever their standard of fitness. If you have not exercised for some time or have had an illness or injury and feel stiff and immobile, you can try these yoga exercises while seated in a chair. Pay particular attention to the breathing and check your positions carefully for the most beneficial results. These exercises are a good substitute for the Sun Salutation and should be done at the same times of day.

Ladder stretch ▶

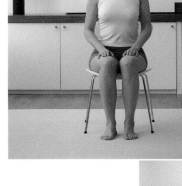

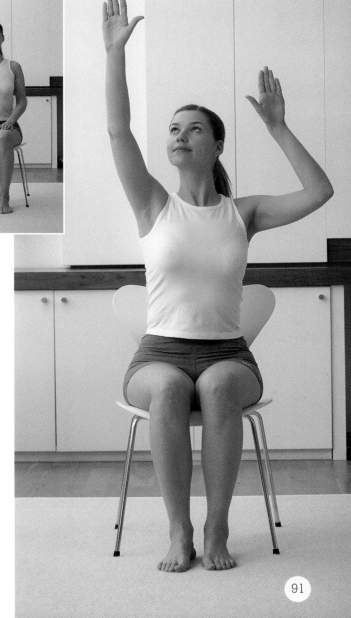

1 Sit on the chair with your feet flat on the floor and a few inches apart. Draw your navel gently in toward your spine so that your back straightens out and any hollow in the small of the back is smoothed away. Although the back is straight, it should be relaxed and the shoulders dropped. Sit in a relaxed position and take three long breaths before you begin, trying to make the inhalation and the exhalation the same length.

2 Breathe in as you stretch your right hand up toward the ceiling, letting the movement come from the shoulder blade, not the top of the shoulder, which should stay dropped. This is not just an arm stretch—you should feel the side of your body stretching, too, with a gap opening between the ribs. Look up at your hand but don't drop your head back.

3 Breathe out as you let your hand drop down to shoulder height, but stay lifted in the body as you do so.

4 Breathe in and stretch the left arm in the same way, and alternate from side to side for as many as ten repetitions, breathing slowly and deeply.

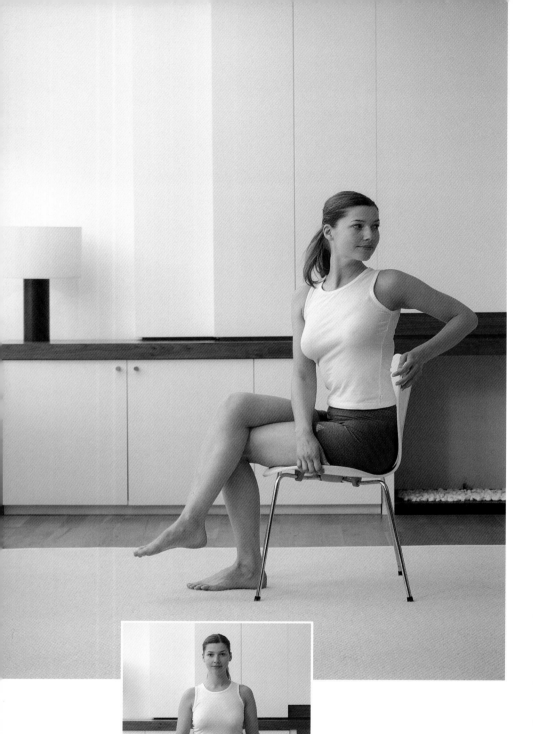

2 Breathe in and, as you breathe out, cross your right leg over the left and start to turn toward your left. The movement should begin at the base of the spine, as if you are revolving around a central pivot. Let the turn gradually ascend up the back, the shoulders, with the head turning last. Don't force the turn in the head, but let it follow the spine naturally.

3 Breathe in and slowly turn back to the center, expanding your lungs as you go. As you breathe out, change your legs so that the left is crossed over the right and turn toward the right in the same way.

4 Alternate from side to side up to ten repetitions, breathing slowly and deeply.

◄**Spinal twist**
1 Sit in the same starting position as in the last exercise, checking again that your navel is drawn in, your back is straight and your shoulders are relaxed.

Forward bend ▶

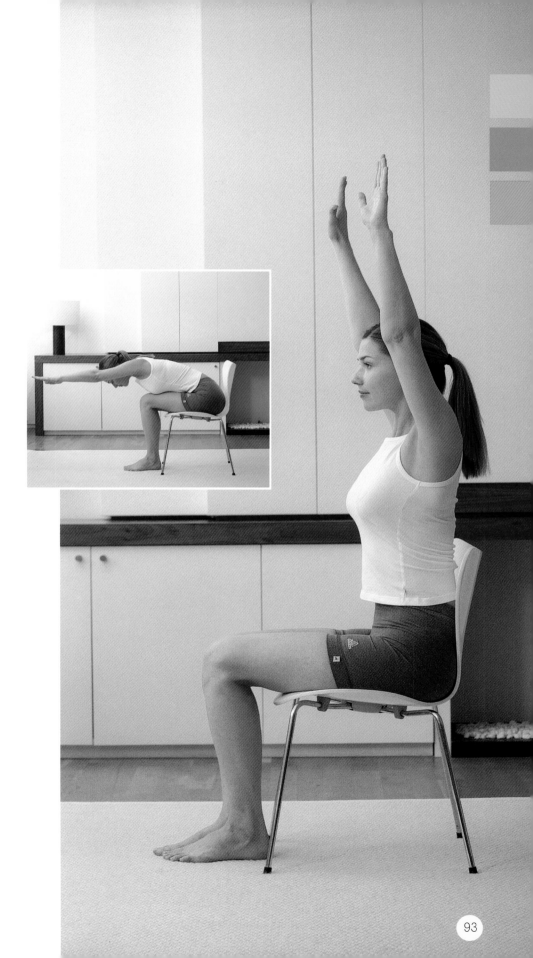

1 Sit on the chair with your feet flat on the floor, the navel gently drawn toward the spine, your back straight and your shoulders dropped. Take a couple of slow, deep breaths.

2 Inhale and stretch both arms up into the air with the movement coming from the shoulder blade rather than lifting the top of the shoulder, which would build tension in the neck and back. Look straight ahead, not at your hands.

3 Exhale slowly and start to drop down toward your legs, arms straight out in front of you and your back straight. This is quite a powerful movement and you need to keep control of your breath and your navel to prevent putting a strain on your back. If this is too strong a movement, drop your arms down to your sides.

4 Inhale and return to the first position. Exhale and begin again for up to ten repetitions.

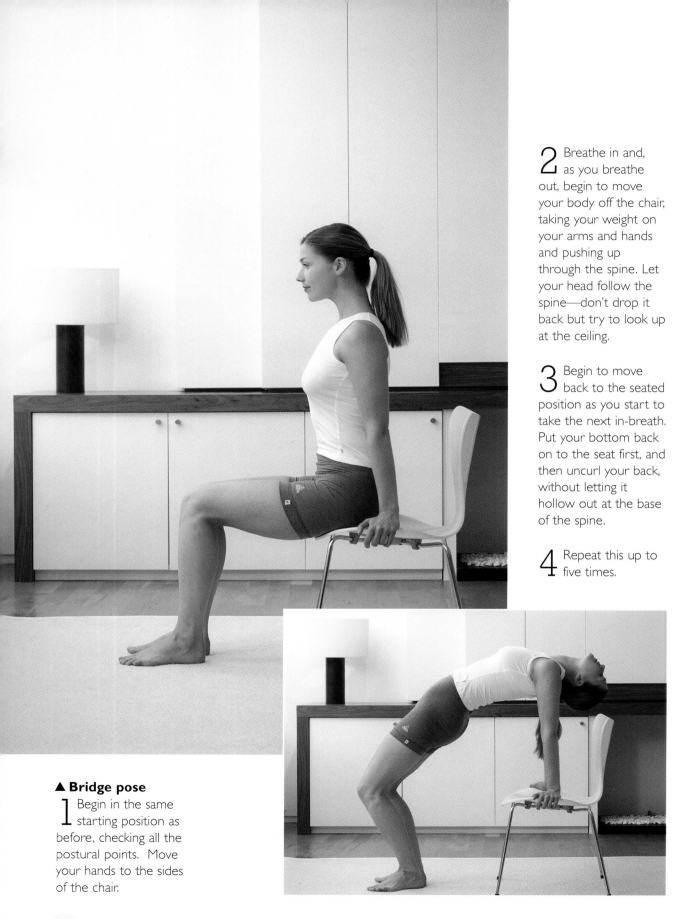

2 Breathe in and, as you breathe out, begin to move your body off the chair, taking your weight on your arms and hands and pushing up through the spine. Let your head follow the spine—don't drop it back but try to look up at the ceiling.

3 Begin to move back to the seated position as you start to take the next in-breath. Put your bottom back on to the seat first, and then uncurl your back, without letting it hollow out at the base of the spine.

4 Repeat this up to five times.

▲ Bridge pose

1 Begin in the same starting position as before, checking all the postural points. Move your hands to the sides of the chair.

▶ Child's pose

1 This is a seated version of the yoga exercise normally done on the floor. Begin in the same starting position as for the other exercises, checking your posture as before. Clasp your hands loosely behind your back.

2 Inhale deeply and, as you exhale, bend forwards until your body is lying along the length of your legs—or as close as you can get to this position. Try to relax into the position and take five long breaths. Return to the starting position.

Rest pose

Sit in the starting position for all of the exercises but with your hands loosely held in your lap. Close your eyes. Breathe deeply and slowly and relax for a few minutes. This is a good pose—and a good time after the stretches to do some breathing exercises such as pranayama (see page 126) or meditation (see page 120–25).

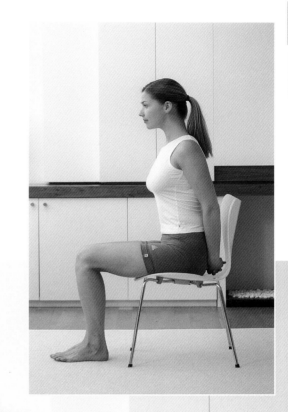

Case history

One couple in their mid-sixties learned yoga at the European ayurveda spa. At first, though they were in good health, they had stiffened up so that they could only manage the Yoga in a Chair exercises. They practiced regularly for six months, by which time they were flexible enough to do the full Sun Salutation and other postures. The beneficial side effects included improvement in their circulation, energy levels, digestion and elimination, and general sense of well-being, so that they felt and looked years younger than their true age.

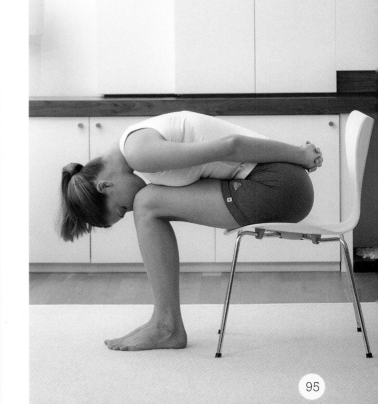

The easy sun salutation

There are several variations on the sun salutation and the first one, shown here, is the easiest to learn and to do. It is a perfect early morning exercise and a good warm-up for other kinds of exercise. It stretches out your whole body and internally massages your organs. Pay special attention to your breathing—this should be the basis on which you build the whole sequence, fitting your movements to your breath rather than the other way around.

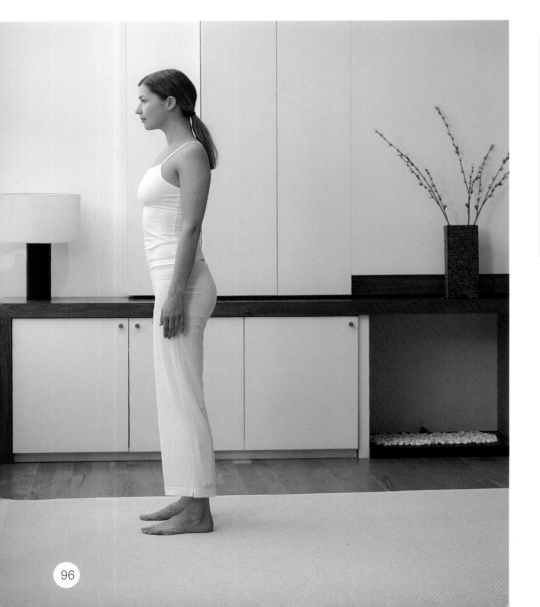

speed

Vatas should follow the sequence slowly, **Pittas** at a moderate speed, **Kaphas** as fast as you can without disturbing your breath. Repeat the sequence between five and ten times.

1 Stand very tall with your navel drawn upward and inward toward the spine, your buttocks tucked under and your back long and straight. Next, hold your hands together in the prayer position, just in front of your breast-bone. Breathe in deeply and exhale two or three times and bring your focus to your breathing and your body.

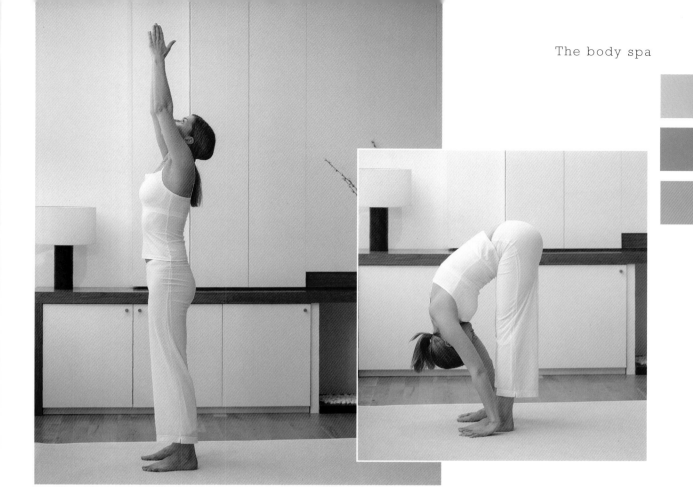

2 Breathe in deeply, stretch your arms above your head and look up at your hands.

3 Exhale, bending forward from the hips with a straight back and arms out-stretched, taking your hands down to the floor, or as close as you can. Your aim is to lay your body along your thighs, but as most people have tight hamstrings you will probably need to bend your knees to do this.

4 Inhale and look up, keeping your hands on the floor.

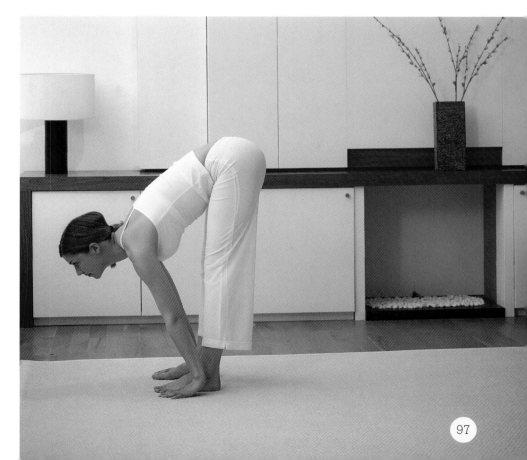

97

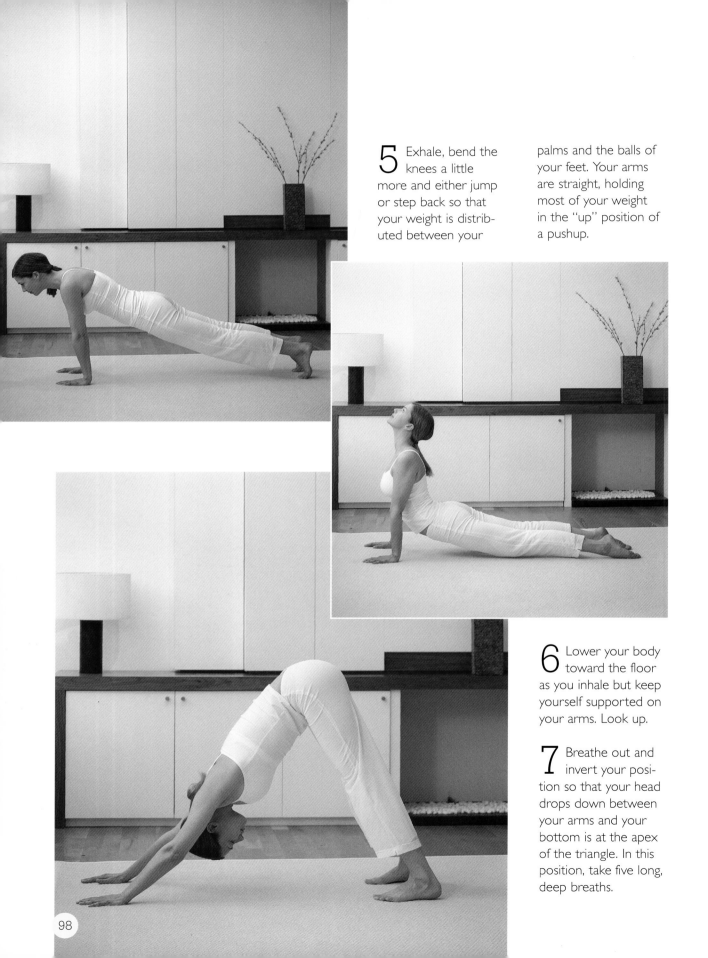

5 Exhale, bend the knees a little more and either jump or step back so that your weight is distributed between your palms and the balls of your feet. Your arms are straight, holding most of your weight in the "up" position of a pushup.

6 Lower your body toward the floor as you inhale but keep yourself supported on your arms. Look up.

7 Breathe out and invert your position so that your head drops down between your arms and your bottom is at the apex of the triangle. In this position, take five long, deep breaths.

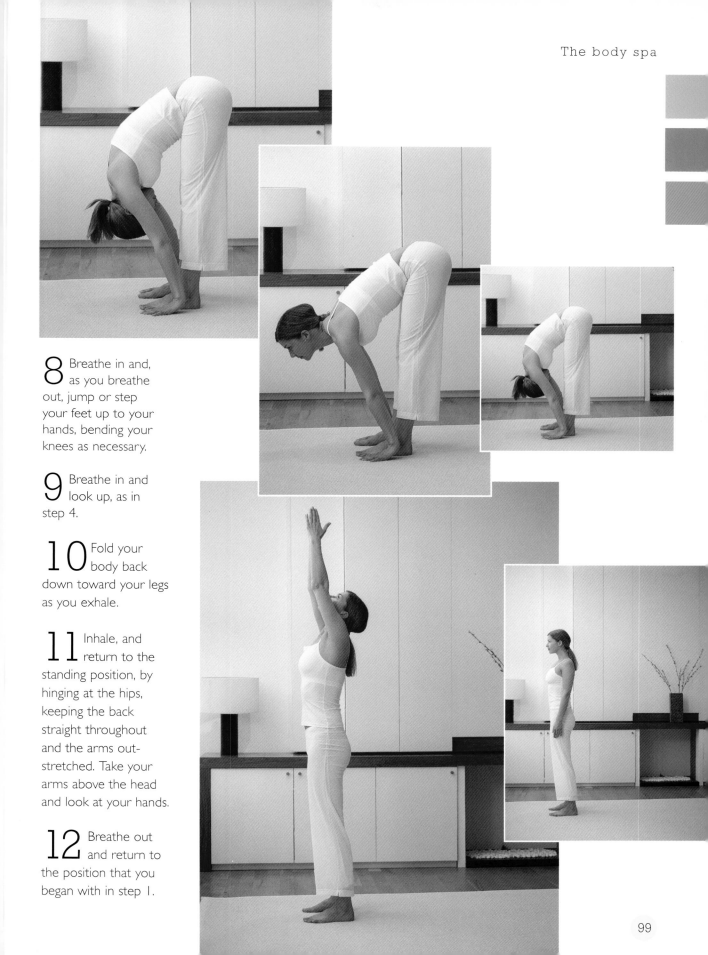

8 Breathe in and, as you breathe out, jump or step your feet up to your hands, bending your knees as necessary.

9 Breathe in and look up, as in step 4.

10 Fold your body back down toward your legs as you exhale.

11 Inhale, and return to the standing position, by hinging at the hips, keeping the back straight throughout and the arms out-stretched. Take your arms above the head and look at your hands.

12 Breathe out and return to the position that you began with in step 1.

Extending the sun salutation

Do not attempt this more complex version of the Sun Salutation until you feel you have completely mastered the easier version together with its rhythmic breathing. This sequence is a longer one than the first and introduces some new poses, but again the most important element is the breathing and you should, once again, let the breath dictate the pace of the movements following it. Ideally, you should do the five repetitions of the easy version and then five repetitions of this one—but build up to this as you get stronger and more supple.

■ Turn to the next pages for a quick visual reference guide to the extended salutation.

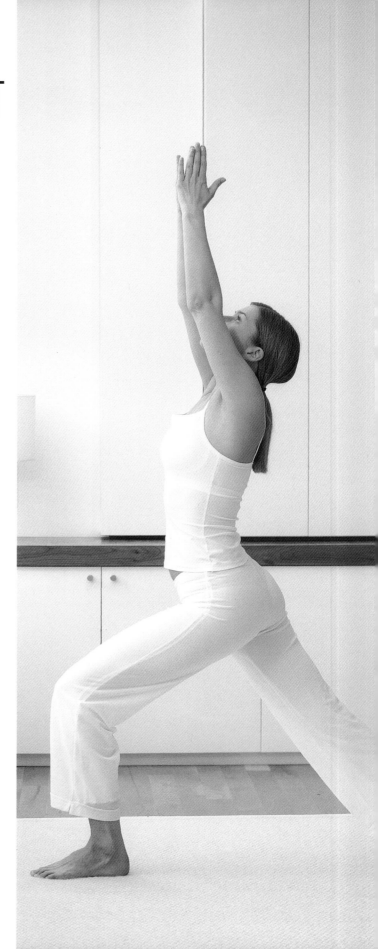

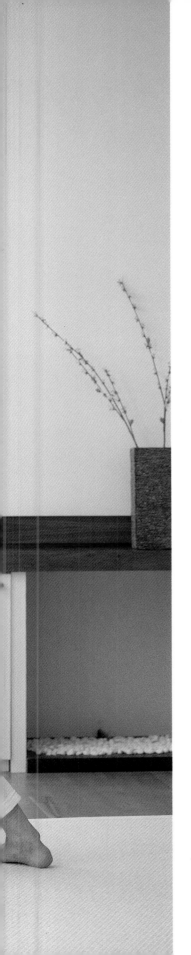

1 Stand very tall with your navel drawn upward and inward toward the spine, your buttocks tucked under and your back long and straight. Next, hold your hands together in the prayer position, just in front of your breastbone. Breathe in deeply and exhale two or three times and bring your focus to your breathing and your body.

2 Breathe in deeply, bend your knees and stretch your arms above your head and look up at your hands.

3 Exhale, bending forward from the hips with a straight back and arms outstretched, taking your hands down to the floor, or as close as you can. Your aim is to lay your body along your thighs, but as most people have tight hamstrings you will probably need to bend your knees to do this.

4 Inhale, and look up, keeping your hands on the floor.

5 Exhale, bend the knees a little more and either jump or step

back so that your weight is distributed between your palms and the balls of your feet. Your arms are straight, holding most of your weight in the "up" position of a pushup.

6 Lower your body toward the floor so that your knees, chest and chin are in contact with the floor, then swing your body up as you inhale, keeping yourself supported on your arms. Look up.

7 Breathe out and invert your position so that your head drops down between your arms and your bottom is at the apex of the triangle.

8 Breathe in, turn your left foot at a right angle and step your right foot up to your hands, bending the right knee, raising your hands above your head and looking up.

9 Breathe out, place your hands back on the floor and step your right foot back to the left one, lowering your body to the floor and repeating step 6.

10 Breathe out and repeat the step 7 triangle.

11 Breathe in, turn your right foot at a right angle and step your left foot up to your hands, bending your left knee, raising your hands above your head and looking up.

12 Breathe out, step your left foot back to meet the right, lower down to the ground and repeat step 6.

13 Breathe out to the inverted triangle of step 7. Take five long, deep breaths.

14 Breathe in and jump the feet forward to the hands. Look up, as in step 4.

15 Fold your body back down toward your legs as you exhale.

16 Breathe in and unfold the body, bending the knees and reaching the hands above the head. Look up.

17 Breathe out and return to the starting position.

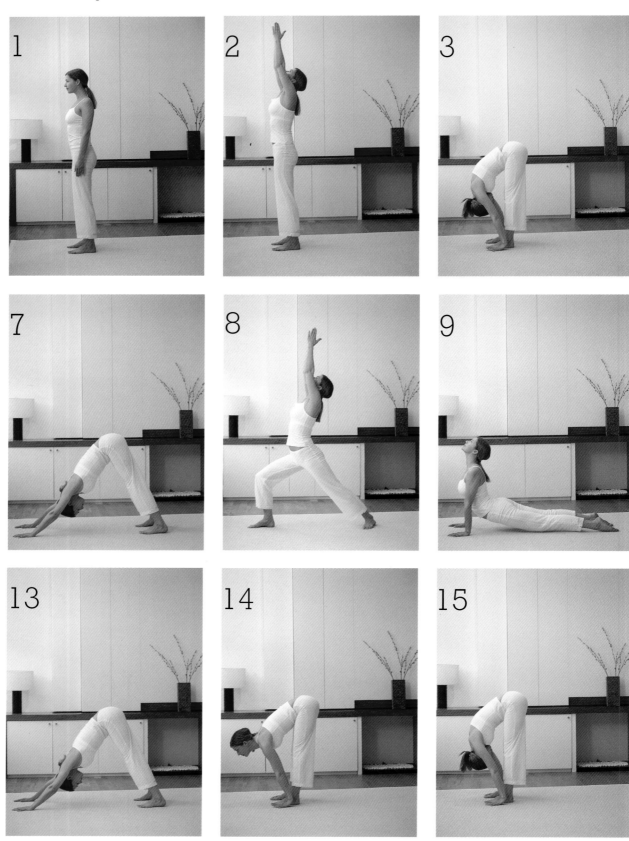

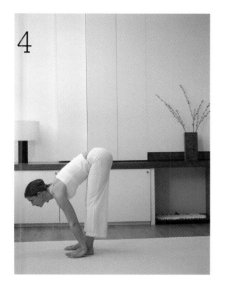

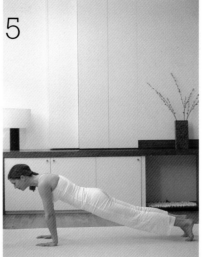

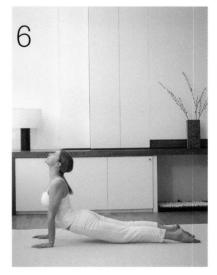

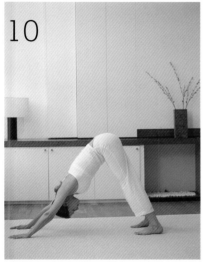

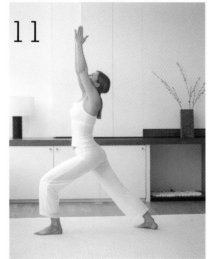

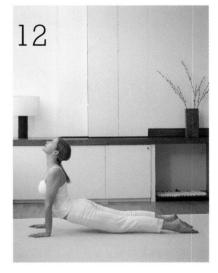

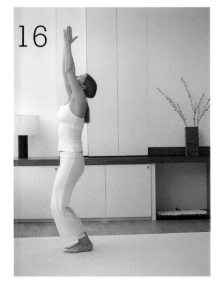

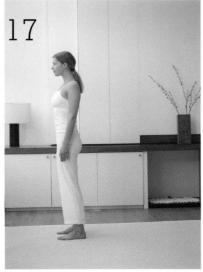

■ Follow the instructions for the extended sun saluta- tion on page 101. Once you are familiar with the sequence you can use the pictures on these pages as a quick visual reference guide.

Yoga postures

Yoga is, of course, a vast and diverse discipline and one that repays years of study, so there is only room to show some of the most popular poses that are appropriate for beginners here. It is always better to learn yoga with an experienced and well-qualified teacher who can help you to improve the way you perform the poses, as well as guiding you through more complex positions and sequences.

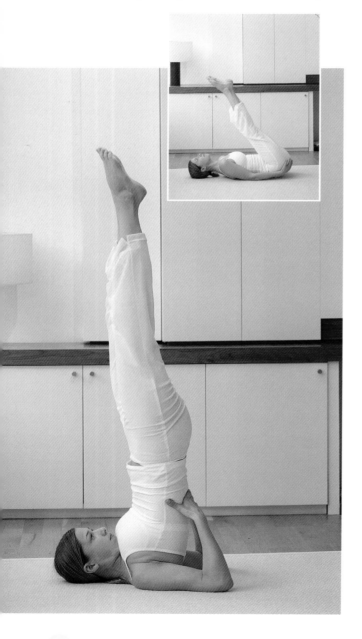

◄ Shoulder stand
This pose is associated with longevity, but should not be performed during menstruation. This pose and the next are believed to improve circulation (specially good for varicose veins), energy and concentration. Do not try to lift your legs all the way up until you have been practicing yoga for a while and do not hold the position for more than a few breaths until you feel comfortable with the pose.

1 Lie flat on the floor with your legs together and your arms at your sides but with a slight gap between them and your body. Take some long, slow breaths and try to relax the spine down on to the floor and lengthen out the neck.

2 Breathe in and bend your knees toward your chest, rolling your hips up from the floor. Place your hands below the hips to support them.

3 If you can, keep raising the legs in one smooth movement until your toes point to the ceiling. If you cannot do this, keep the legs bent.

4 In this position, take some long, slow breaths, straightening your back and pressing your chin on to your chest—this stimulates the thyroid and parathyroid glands, which, it is suggested, will delay aging.

5 Follow the same sequence of movements on the way down and rest, breathing deeply, in the corpse pose (see page 107).

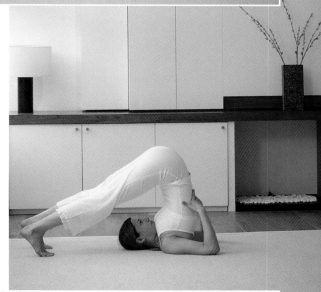

drop them down to the floor. When you feel comfortable in this position, you can flex the feet back so they are "on the walk" with the toes curled under—this will increase the stretch. When you are in position, close your eyes and take five or more long, slow breaths.

4 To come out of the pose, raise your legs, drop your knees down to your chest and roll the spine down slowly, finally stretching your legs out along the floor and resting in the corpse pose.

The plough ▶
This pose is very similar to the last one and you can alternate between them.

1 Lie flat on the floor with your legs together and your arms at your sides but with a slight gap between them and your body. Take some long, slow breaths and try to relax the spine down on to the floor and lengthen out the neck.

2 Breathe in and bend your knees toward your chest, rolling your hips up from the floor. Place your hands below the hips to support them.

3 Breathing out, point your toes behind your head and, supporting the back with the hands, let the feet go beyond the head and, if you can,

105

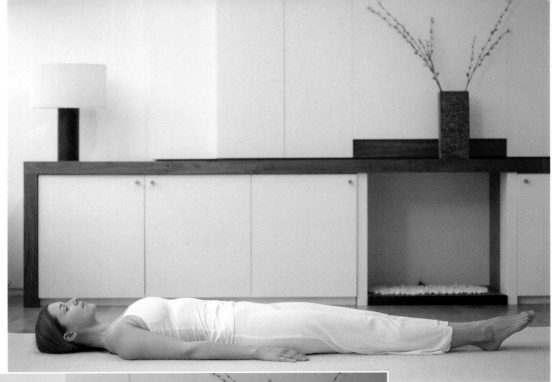

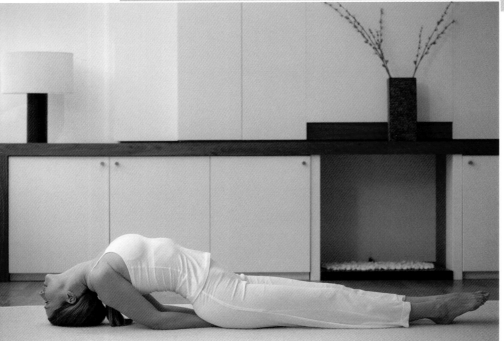

▲ The fish

This pose bends the body in the opposite way to the shoulder stand, opening out the chest, and is a good way of balancing the positions. Do not do this position if you have neck problems.

If you suffer from hypertension, do not put your head on the floor in step 2, as there is a vital pressure point at the top of the head. Instead, bend your head back until it is about an inch from the floor.

1 Lie on your back with your legs together, stretched out in front of you, your toes pointing away. Breathe in and begin to arch your back from the floor.

2 Breathe out and slide your hands under your buttocks. With bent elbows and the lower arms on the floor, support your upper body. Arch up so that the back is curved and the top of your head rests on the floor. Hold this position while you take several deep breaths.

3 Slide the back of your head, your neck and then your back down to the floor. Relax for a few moments.

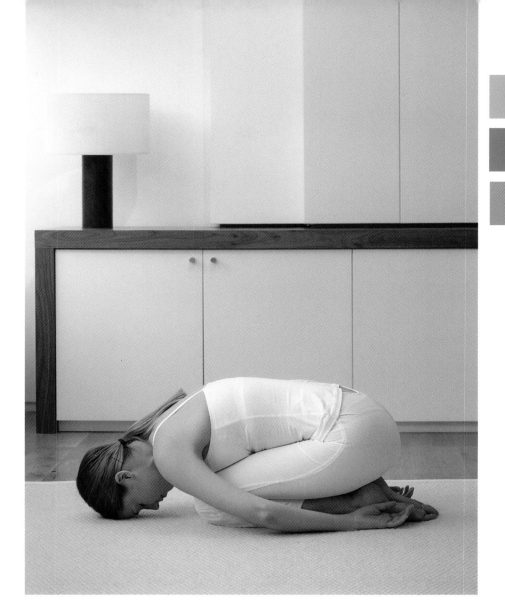

▶ Child's pose

This is a good pose for relaxation after a yoga session, specially if your back is not used to so much stretching.

1 Sit on your heels, keeping your back straight. Place your hands on the soles of your feet. Breathe in and bend gently backwards, looking up.

2 Breathe out and bend forwards until you can place your forehead on the floor. You will have to let go of your feet and your bottom may come up a little. Let your arms rest against your sides and breathe slowly and deeply for a few minutes with your eyes closed. If you prefer, you can turn your head to the side.

3 Bring your breathing back to normal and sit up very slowly.

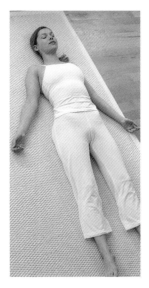

◀ The corpse pose

This pose is so relaxing that you might find yourself falling asleep and you should do it at the end of your session. Make sure you have something to cover yourself with or you may begin to feel cold.

1 Lie on your back with your arms slightly away from your sides, the palms facing upward. Your legs should be slightly apart, with the feet relaxed, the toes facing out. Close your eyes.

2 Breathe slowly and deeply for one or two minutes, concentrating on the breath itself and the sensation of the air in your lungs. Bring your breath back to normal for a few minutes before you get up.

The vata daily routine

Vata's elements are air and ether and vata is the dosha of ideas—with a creative and imaginative mind. When out of balance, however, Vatas are restless and unsettled, constantly blown from one idea, place or project to the next. To feel settled, Vatas need grounding and the best way to do this is by establishing a daily routine—though Vatas will find any routine much harder to adhere to than either of the other two doshas. Nevertheless, this will help Vatas to maintain focus and energy levels, and prevent anxiety and stress.

Main priorities for
balance

- Practice meditation, yoga or balanced breathing twice a day
- Give yourself an oil massage once a day
- Have a regular routine of eating and sleeping

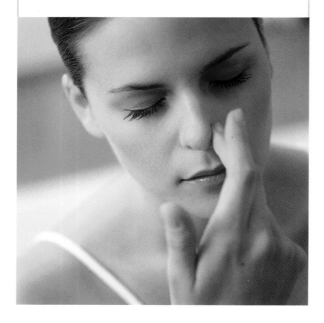

One of Vata people's qualities is coldness and so Vatas crave warmth and comfort. The daily routine for Vatas therefore hinges on providing a regular rhythm for the day that is soothing, warming and nourishing—a sound base for Vatas' creativity and enthusiasm. Cold weather, especially wind, plays havoc with vata and so you should always wrap up well in winter, protecting the head and ears in particular.

The cold, dry qualities that characterize vata need to be balanced by warm, sweet, oily foods (see pages 56–7) and you should eat regular meals in a calm environment, with your attention focussed on your food. Try to avoid the Vata inclination to read, listen to the radio or work while eating.

Because Vatas have a tendency to over-activity, there is an equal tendency to run out of energy and accumulate fatigue within the system. For this reason, only light exercise is recommended (see page 88).

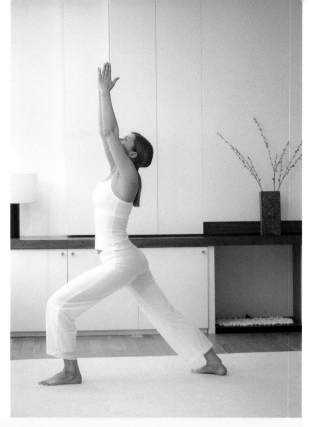

The daily cycle

A.M.	■ Get up before 7 A.M.—6 A.M. ideally—drink a cup of hot water, evacuate bowels. ■ Oil self-massage (see page 134–7) using sesame oil on the body, coconut oil on the head in hot weather and sunflower or olive oil in cold weather. ■ Sun Salutation (see pages 96–103) for a couple of minutes, building up to ten minutes. ■ Shower, scrape tongue (see page 69) and clean teeth. ■ Ten minutes of yoga, followed by two to three minutes of balanced breathing. ■ Five minutes of meditation, building up to twenty minutes.
A.M.	■ A light breakfast, toast with ghee and jam, morning energy drink or camomile tea.
NOON	■ Twenty to thirty minutes before lunch, take ginger pickle. Lunch to be the largest and heaviest meal of the day.
P.M.	■ After lunch, sit comfortably (or lie down) for five minutes and then take a gentle ten-minute walk.
P.M.	■ Mid-afternoon (around 3 P.M.) take a quiet break for ten minutes, listen to soothing calming music, drink an herbal tea, or—if you feel under par—have a cup of the morning energy drink to boost energy and soothe the nervous system.
P.M.	■ Repeat yoga, pranayama and meditation in the late afternoon or early evening.
P.M.	■ Finish your evening meal by 7 P.M. (or as early as you can). Eat lightly—soup, rice, noodles, toast—preceded by ginger pickle, as at lunchtime.
P.M.	■ Be in bed by 10 P.M.

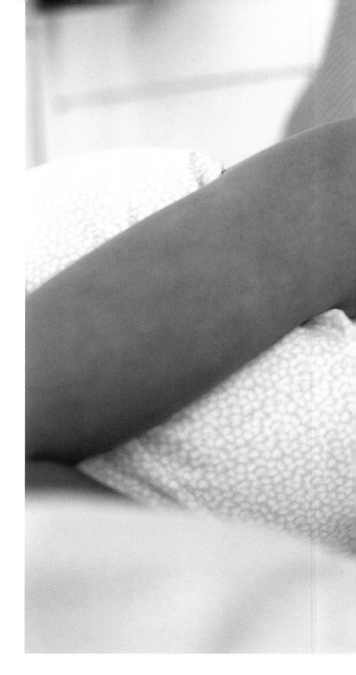

Sleep routine

Vatas' excitable minds do not usually fall naturally into a deep sleep, but without a sound, restorative night's rest Vatas will be unfocussed and lacking in energy the next day. The key to establishing a good sleep pattern is, as with most things for Vatas, a matter of the right routine.

You should start preparing for the night during the course of the evening by settling the mind. Anything that is overstimulating should be avoided after 8.30 P.M.—conversation, films, radio, television, books and, above all, work. All of these activities will keep the mind too active and interfere with your sleep.

The second kapha phase of the day is from 6 P.M. to 10 P.M. and during this period you may start to feel drowsy. In fact, Vatas benefit greatly from going to bed by 10 P.M. whenever possible and sleep begun before then is often particularly deep, making it less likely to be broken during the night. This is due to soft, deep kapha qualities of this period that govern your sleep. In addition, if you are asleep during the pitta phase that follows from 10 P.M. to 2 A.M., your body will be better able to repair and renew itself on a cellular level, ready for the next day.

Other ways to promote sleep include the bedtime drink (see page 62) or a relaxing herbal infusion, such as camomile or lemon verbena, and using lavender or rose essential oil in a burner or just pouring two or three drops on to your pillow. A short meditation of up to twenty minutes earlier in the evening will also help to calm the mind. Finally, do not worry if sleep still does not come quickly. Just being in bed—especially before 10 P.M.—with your eyes closed will be beneficial in itself.

Vata balancing activities

■ Walking in sheltered natural surroundings, especially in moonlight
■ Walking barefoot in warm weather
■ Tai Chi
■ Yoga
■ A little red wine in the evening
■ Alternate-nostril breathing technique (see page 126), especially if you notice your breathing is shallow

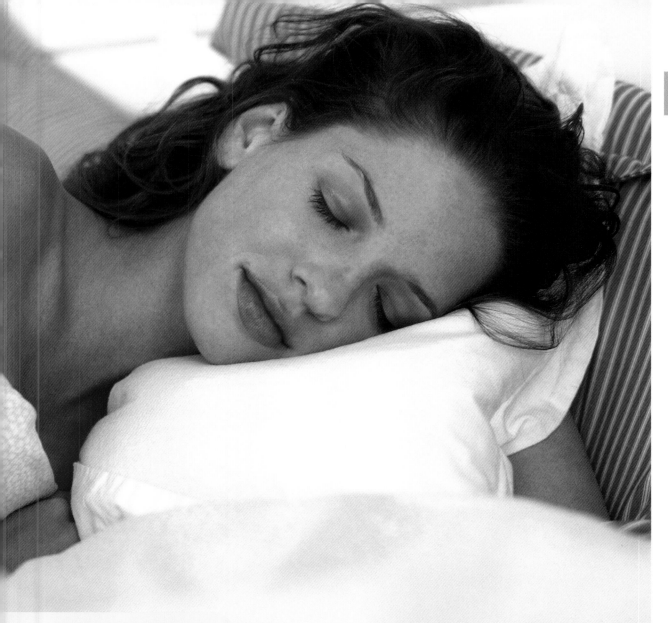

Case history

Vata-pitta Sleep Problems

One couple in their mid-forties had an enviably happy marriage—with one drawback. In the middle of the night (2–3 A.M.), the wife would wake up feeling cold, anxious and lonely. When her husband woke the next morning, he would feel hot, irritable and grumpy. The Vata wife needed more rest and would go to bed before her husband, ensuring the bedroom was warm and free from drafts. When her Pitta husband went to bed, the room would be too hot and stuffy for him, so he would open the windows and turn off the heating. When she woke in the night, she would close the windows and turn the heating on again, so that her husband would wake up an overheated Pitta. The solution was to change the bedroom around so that the husband slept by the window while the wife slept by the radiators, they bought a split-tog duvet with the heavier, warmer side for the wife, and they compromised on the room temperature.

The pitta daily routine

Pitta's elements are fire and water, but it is fire that predominates. Pittas tend to be fiery by nature. You can be passionate, a true champion of strongly held convictions; you will argue fiercely with your incisive, penetrating intellect. However, when you are out of balance, you can become irritable, impatient and aggressive, and your fine organizational skills can become controlling.

Main priorities for **balance**

- Eat a satisfying lunch every day, favoring organic, unprocessed, pitta-pacifying foods
- Keep your body cool
- Never skip any meal

Physically as well as mentally Pittas are fiery. Pitta governs the body's metabolism, in particular the way it digests food, and it is essential for Pittas to eat regular, satisfying meals. If they skip lunch the entire afternoon will be upset. It is always better to approach Pittas with a thorny problem after they have had a large, satisfying lunch, when their mood will be mellow and the formidable Pitta intellect will be at its sharpest. Approach a hungry Pitta at your peril!

On every level, then, Pittas need to be cooled down. Try to make your living and working place airy and spacious and the temperature low. Sitting in the sun or hot environments should be avoided whenever possible. Don't wear yourself out with competitive sports—your favorite form of exercise —moderate, regular exercise is better. All forms of competition increase pitta—think of John McEnroe under pressure. Strenuous exercise also makes you hot—something, of course, you should be trying to avoid. Swimming is the perfect, cooling way for Pittas to exercise (see also page 89).

Regular meals are absolutely essential for Pittas, lunch being particularly important—and it must be eaten slowly. Eating quickly is a Pitta tendency that often results in acidity, heartburn and indigestion. Pittas tend to gulp down food; this habit can be overriden by always putting down your fork between mouthfuls. You will need to think about this at first, but eventually you will start to do it naturally. You need to eat sweet, bitter, heavy and cooling foods (see pages 58–9) to avoid stomach acid, indigestion—and bad moods! If you are upset, you should wait until you feel calmer before you eat, and you should always try to take your meals in a friendly, settled environment, giving the food all your attention and really enjoying it. You should not overeat, though. After a main meal, the stomach should be between half and two-thirds full. When you have finished, sit still for five minutes and relax.

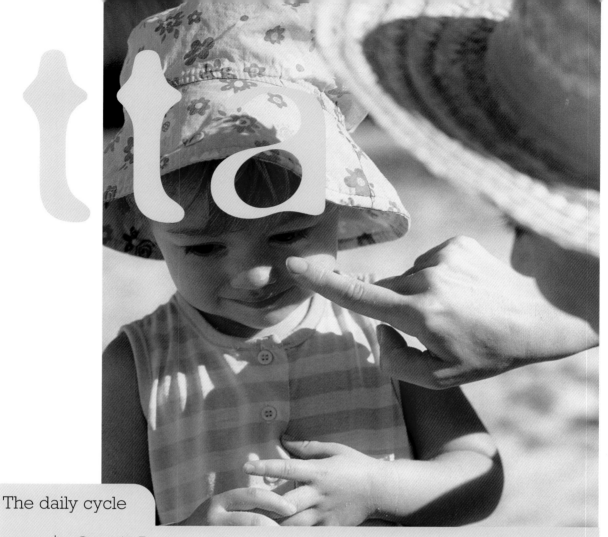

The daily cycle

A.M.	■ Get up by 7 A.M. ■ Drink a cup of hot water, evacuate bowels. ■ Oil massage, using coconut oil if you feel too warm, rather than sesame oil (see pages 134–7). ■ Sun Salutation for five to ten minutes (see pages 96–103).
A.M.	■ Shower, scrape tongue (see page 69). ■ Yoga for ten minutes, balanced breathing for two to three minutes.
A.M.	■ Meditation for twenty minutes.
A.M.	■ Light breakfast, toast with ghee and jam, morning energy drink or peppermint tea. Drinks should be room temperature—avoid iced drinks.
NOON	■ Eat lunch as close to midday as possible. Lunch should be the most substantial meal of the day.
P.M.	■ Repeat the yoga, breathing techniques and meditation in the early evening.
P.M.	■ Be in bed by 10 P.M.

Sleep routine

Pittas sleep soundly but do not need a particularly long sleep to feel refreshed the next day. Like Vatas, you should start preparing for the night during the course of the evening by settling the mind. Anything that is overstimulating should be avoided after 8.30 P.M.—conversation, films, radio, books and television.

The second kapha phase of the day is from 6 P.M. to 10 P.M. and during this period you may start to feel drowsy; by going to bed by 10 P.M. you will have a particularly restorative sleep. During the pitta phase that follows from 10 P.M. to 2 A.M. your body will repair and renew itself, ready for the next day.

Pitta hair care

Excess pitta has a direct effect on hair, causing premature graying and hair loss by burning the hair follicles and stripping minerals as it goes. Generally, anything that lowers pitta can help, so following the daily routine will boost hair health naturally. Other hair remedies include:

■ Massage your scalp with coconut oil—rich in calcium and cooling for Pittas
■ Avoid using sesame oil on your scalp (see self-massage page 134–7) as its heating quality is inappropriate here
■ Gently comb your hair in the opposite direction to its growth, to increase circulation to the roots, avoiding vigorous strokes as this will cause further damage
■ Eat more coconut, coconut milk and dairy products (except for very strong cheese, which is pitta-aggravating) as they lower pitta and also contain calcium
■ Drink a third of a tea cup of aloe vera juice daily
■ White radish, almonds and a daily handful of white sesame seeds are beneficial
■ Amla fruit, the main ingredient in Chawanprash (available from Indian health food shops), is very nourishing
■ 1200 mg calcium, 600 mg magnesium and 60 mg zinc mineral supplements taken at bedtime are also beneficial

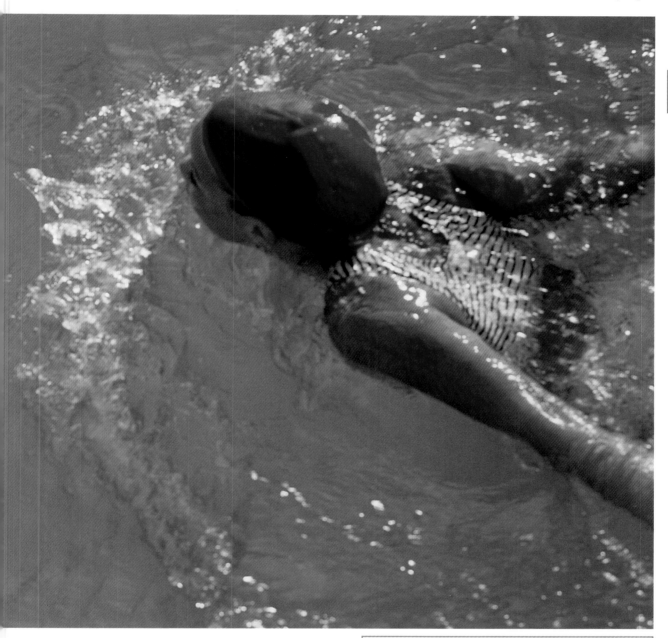

Swimming or walking in beautiful scenery is a great pitta balancing activity.

Pitta **balancing** activities

- Doing anything in a cool, spacious environment
- Walking in beautiful scenery—by water if at all possible
- Skiing
- Swimming
- Moderate, non-competitive exercise

The kapha daily routine

Kapha's elements are earth and water, earth being dominant, and it is this that gives Kaphas strength and stamina. Kapha is the most stable of the doshas, slow to rouse to anger and both patient and compassionate. However, without sufficient stimulation, Kaphas become slow and sluggish and mentally dull.

Kaphas have a slow metabolism and a tendency to gain weight and so need to take more—and more vigorous—exercise than the other doshas. Exercise also helps to keep Kaphas mentally alert, especially if you choose a sport or exercise that requires quick reactions and fast thinking. For a clear mind and a productive day, Kaphas need to get up early and exercise straight away—despite your natural inclination to stay in bed! You have the deepest sleep of all of the doshas but, if you have too much sleep (again your natural tendency) it will slow you down.

Your calmness, strength and steadfastness are considerable virtues, but if kapha goes out of balance you will get stuck in a rut. The best way to keep kapha on its toes and to keep lethargy at bay is to give yourself challenges and make frequent changes.

Kaphas need protection against cold and damp. Make sure you keep warm (especially your head and chest) in winter and avoid mucus-forming foods (ice cream, hard cheese, cold milk, cold or fatty foods in general). Kapha, for all its strength, has the weakest digestion of all the body types, since it lacks fire or movement and, without sufficient digestive stimulus, produces excess mucus at all times. (Never swallow mucus.)

Sleep routine

Kaphas fall naturally into a heavy sleep. Nevertheless, avoid anything that is overstimulating after 8.30 P.M.—conversation, films, radio, books and television. Go to bed by 10 P.M. and you will have a particularly restorative sleep.

Main priorities for **balance**

■ Get up early each morning and exercise vigorously every day
■ Take ginger pickle before every meal (see page 62)
■ Do the unexpected—step outside your normal boundaries!

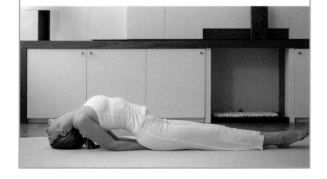

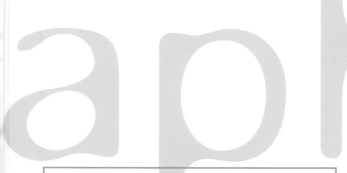

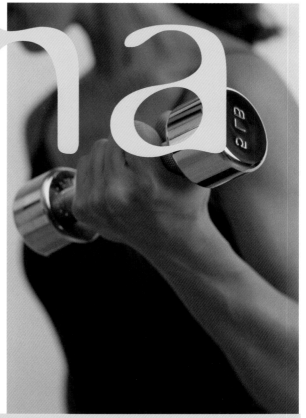

Kapha **balancing** activities

■ Running
■ Circuit-training
■ Heavy gardening
■ Any sport that involves fast movement and thinking
■ Any new, challenging activity

The daily cycle

A.M.	■ Get up before 7 A.M. ■ Drink a cup of hot water or fresh coffee if it's cold outside, evacuate bowels. ■ Dry massage, with bare hands or raw silk gloves (see page 133). ■ Sun Salutation for five to ten minutes (see pages 96–103).
A.M.	■ Vigorous exercise for about half an hour.
A.M.	■ Shower, scrape tongue (see page 69). ■ Yoga for ten minutes, balanced breathing for two to three minutes.
A.M.	■ Meditation for twenty minutes. ■ Skip breakfast if you are not hungry. Otherwise eat very lightly and drink hot spicy herbal tea.
NOON	■ Eat lunch as close to midday as possible. Lunch should be the most substantial meal of the day.
P.M.	■ Repeat the yoga, breathing techniques and meditation in the early evening.
P.M.	■ Eat very lightly in the evening, taking ginger pickle beforehand.
P.M.	■ Be in bed by 10 P.M.

Chapter six

The mind spa

Yoga is often thought of as purely physical exercise, but it is much more than this. When practiced regularly, it leaves you feeling invigorated—both mentally and physically—and calm. It becomes, in effect, a form of moving meditation, though this can only be achieved when your attention is devoted to what you are doing. Distractions will detract from the benefits of yoga, and it is better to do your practice in silence and, if possible, at the same time each day. The rhythms of the repeated sequences help to achieve a state of mindfulness, where the focus is purely on the here and now, your breath and your body. This is a perfect preparation for the meditation that we explore in this chapter. The basis of both yoga and meditation is this integration of the mind and the body in a state of pure consciousness. Meditation is often regarded by Westerners as an entirely foreign concept that involves contorting your body into bizarre positions or isolating yourself from the world. European ayurveda does not see it in this way, but rather as the perfect antidote to stress in a high-pressure world. Just as the body spa showed you how to give yourself a healthier, more relaxed body, the mind spa shows you a simple but effective way of achieving a natural state of calm.

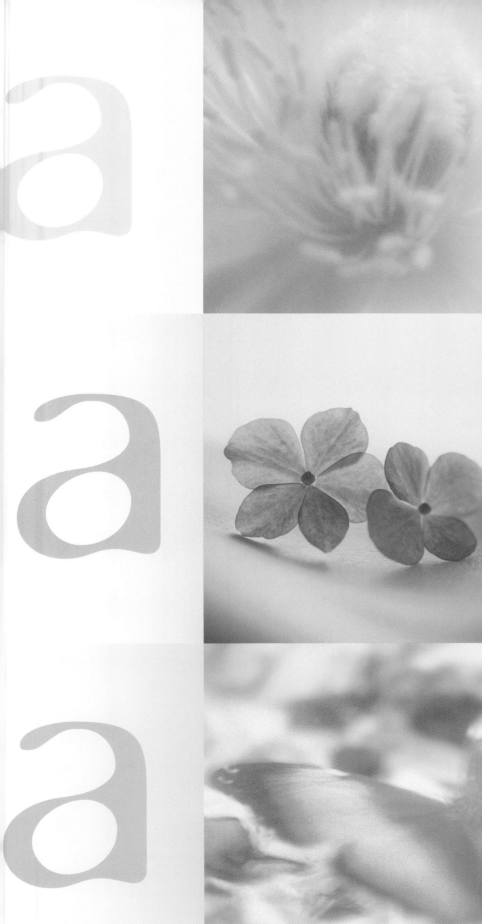

Vata people

Meditation:
ten minutes in the
morning, after your
yoga, and again in
the late afternoon
or early evening

Pitta people

Meditation:
twenty minutes in
the morning, after
your yoga, and again
in the early evening

Kapha people

Meditation:
twenty minutes in
the morning, after
your yoga, and again
in the late afternoon
or early evening

Meditation

The last hundred years have seen unprecedented scientific advances beyond the wildest dreams of previous generations, with much of the physical hardship of life eradicated (at least in the West) and a hugely improved standard of living. They ushered in a time of relentless change, speed and innovation, and as we race to keep up we are faced—in place of the old fatal infectious diseases we have wiped out—with new killer illnesses that are often the direct result of the stress and anxiety that are now an everyday part of life.

European ayurveda's solution to stress is meditation, using a very simple technique to create a settled mind, a feeling of inner peace and, as a direct result of these, an improved lifestyle often without many of the habits that were a cause of stress in the first place.

Meditation first came to the notice of the West in the 1960s, when the Beatles amongst others went to India to learn the technique from the Maharishi Mahesh Yogi. Dismissed as an Eastern fad for hippies at first, meditation is nowadays used all over the world by people of every age and background for its calming and relaxing effects, while in business many major companies have found that it boosts productivity and reduces days lost by sickness. It is this form of transcendental meditation using a mantra that is recommended by European ayurveda.

Effortless bliss

Many people are put off the idea of learning to meditate because of its Eastern origins, assuming that they will have to accept a new belief system or a change of lifestyle. In fact, while Eastern philosophies provide an endlessly rich source of study, European ayurveda teaches both transcendental

meditation and pranayama as straightforward techniques, resulting in lowered stress levels and improved physical and mental well-being.

No special postures are required—you can just sit comfortably in a chair with your eyes closed while you meditate—because you should be in a state of deep rest and relaxation. The key to meditation is that the mind is naturally still. You do not force it into a state of concentration, but allow it to rest in silence.

The wandering mind

Many people assume, however, that they will not be able to meditate because, far from their minds resting in silence, they would be bored and fidget and find their minds wandering off on to inconsequential ideas. "Where am I going tomorrow?" "Have I fed the cat?" "What do I have to do when I've finished meditating?" However, according to European ayurveda, it is inevitable the mind will wander—but that does not mean you will not be able to meditate.

Having an active mind does not mean that it cannot be still. That would be rather like looking at the sea and saying that it is rough when you are judging it only by its surface. If you were to dive into

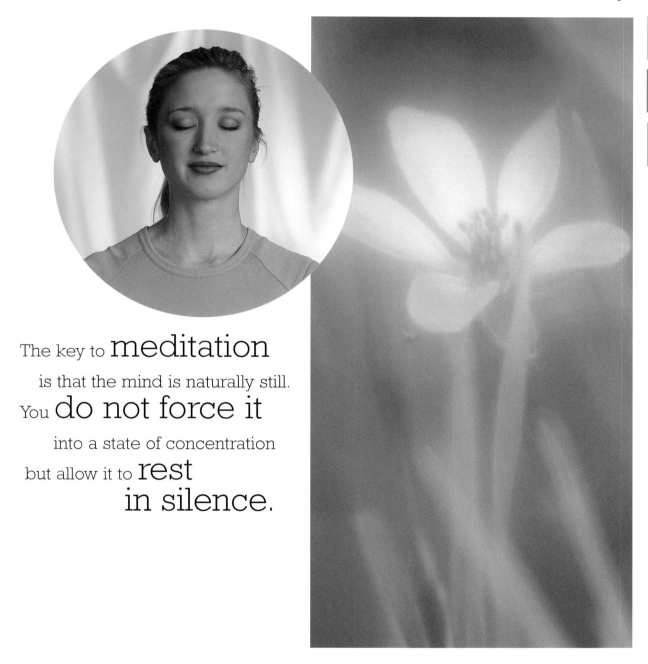

The key to **meditation** is that the mind is naturally still. You **do not force it** into a state of concentration but allow it to **rest in silence.**

the sea, you would find that, the lower you went, the more still it became. Without its underlying, silent depths the waves above would not exist. Scientists express this as "the excited state contains the less excited state." In other words, any organism in nature capable of activity can also be less active and ultimately totally still. Your mind is no exception. If you can run, you can stop running. If you can think, you can stop thinking.

In fact, when the mind wanders, it goes in search of a state of happiness—just as all our actions, whether planning a holiday, buying a house or car, changing career or embarking on a relationship, have this same underlying aim. Where the mind finds happiness is not, though, on a sun-baked beach or in a new Porsche, but in an underlying ocean of consciousness: a blissful silent state that is its true nature.

121

During **meditation**, the mind turns its attention away from **sensory** experience … to **mental** experience … until even **thinking** fades away and all that is left is "I am."

According to European ayurveda, our thoughts—appearing apparently randomly and constantly every waking moment of our lives—begin as an impulse in the unconscious mind, rising like a bubble to the surface. This represents a tiny part of our minds' potential, though. According to the scientists, we are using less than 10 percent of the mind (some say as little as 0.1 percent). When we dive deeper than this surface level and experience during meditation more subtle levels of mental activity, we expand the capacity of the conscious mind—as has been shown in the heightened creativity and mental performance of meditators (see below).

During meditation, the mind turns its attention away from sensory experience ("I am doing") to mental experience ("I am thinking") until even thinking fades away and all that is left is "'I am." This peaceful, serene state is simply the experience of our own inner being, beyond suffering and negative thinking. As children, we were not cynical or depressed and such negative emotions are not natural to us. Rather, they are the products of accumulated stress. We were born without them. We can be without them again.

Natural intelligence

When we reach this ocean of consciousness during meditation, our minds are not—as is often thought—empty. Quite the reverse. We are experiencing the infinite creativity and intelligence of nature itself, and of our own true nature, which is a part of it. Whether you consider the vastness of galaxies or a single snowflake, evidence of nature's harmonious creative intelligence is all around us.

Our own bodies are one such remarkable example. Millions of biochemical impulses take place in the human body every second. The healing process itself—even in such a minor case as a cut finger—entails thousands of intricate and delicately balanced procedures we cannot begin to replicate artificially. We have our own internal pharmacies, capable of making all the drugs needed to keep in balance—tranquillizers, anti-depressants, sleeping pills, antibiotics and anti-cancer drugs—all without side effects and delivered in the right dose, at the right time and in the right place. Much of this knowledge of our bodies is newly discovered, but our bodies' natural intelligence has been employing it since the dawn of our evolutionary time. When we meditate, we access this natural intelligence and this results in a vast range of well-documented benefits. A study of health insurance statistics for 2,000 people practicing meditation over a five-year period showed they had consistently less than half the doctor visits and hospitalization of other groups of comparable age, gender, profession and insurance terms. Significantly, the differences increased with age—so older meditators required even less treatment than non-meditators. In particular, the meditators had 87 percent less hospitalization for heart disease, 55 percent less for cancer, 87 percent less for disorders of the nervous system and 73 percent less for nose, throat and lung problems.

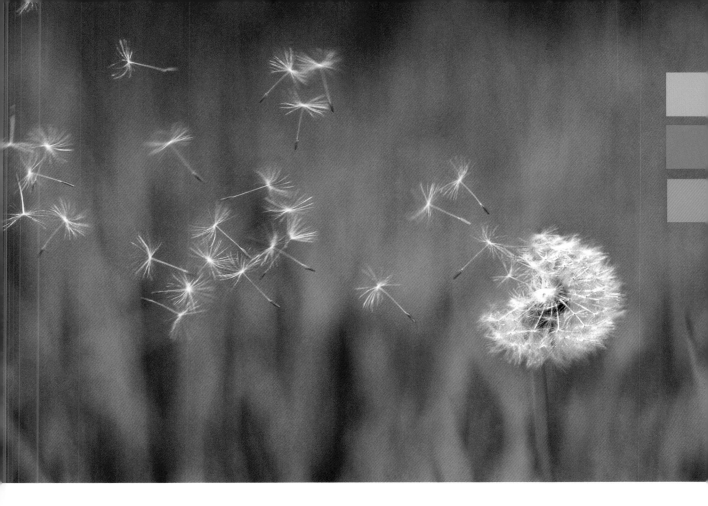

The benefits of meditation

Over the last thirty years there have been many clinical research studies into the benefits of regular transcendental meditation. Interestingly, these benefits have been shown to begin immediately—and despite any skepticism on the part of the meditator—and to continue throughout the day after the meditation itself has finished.

Enhanced brain performance

As the mind becomes accustomed to more subtle, intuitive levels of thinking, brain-wave activity becomes orderly and coherent. Electroencephalograph (EEG) tests show that electrical waves produced during meditation are different than those we produce at other times, whether asleep or awake. Electrical activity takes on a slow rhythm, with regular, even waves recorded from different parts of the brain. This regularity continues after meditation, too, with sustained practice. Alpha and Theta waves, indicating a rest-

fully alert state, appear in the central and rear areas of the cortex and then spread toward the frontal lobes, a phenomenon otherwise rarely seen. The left and right hemispheres of the brain become highly synchronized in their activity and the brain's information-processing systems become finely tuned. This coherent brain activity is, according to medical research, seen to be present in improved mental performance, such as increased creativity and intelligence, problem-solving and decision-making, better memory and learning ability, mental clarity, comprehension, concentration and reaction time. Such improvements naturally result in increased self-confidence and self-esteem, reduced anxiety and depression, and reduced use of alcohol, cigarettes and drugs.

Deep physical rest

When the mind settles during meditation, the body's stress levels reduce too. Breathing becomes shallower, the heart rate slows down and the whole cardiovascular system gains very deep rest. The blood pressure lowers and the respiratory rate slows, but the same levels of oxygen remain in the blood. Circulation improves and activity in the autonomic nervous system reduces. The levels of various chemicals that occur naturally in the body and are indicative of stress, such as blood lactate and cortisol, are significantly reduced, while other life-supporting chemicals, such as plasma prolactin and phenylalanine, increase. Tense muscles automatically relax, tension and fatigue are reduced, the immune system is strengthened and cholesterol is reduced. Other side-effects of this deep rest commonly include relief from or reduction of headaches, migraines, asthma, panic attacks, eczema, psoriasis, irritable bowel syndrome, diabetes, PMS and coronary heart disease.

Improved sports performance and relationships

Just as stress negatively affects every aspect of life, the practice of meditation, by dissolving the stress, improves it. Sporting performance, job performance and productivity all commonly improve. Many meditators report that personal relationships also become more harmonious when stress ebbs away.

Reduced cancer risk

Research is still going on into whether meditation can have any effect on cancer. Certain types of cancer are thought to appear at times of great stress, because stress can damage the functioning of the immune system, which is needed to destroy cancer cells. Diminishing stress by meditation is therefore thought by some practitioners to have a place in cancer treatment, though as yet there has not been sufficient research to judge.

How meditation works

Vedic science—the profound knowledge that forms the basis of ayurveda—is uncannily akin to modern quantum physics. In quantum physics, the study of sub-atomic particles has revealed that the most basic constituents of creation, including ourselves, do not consist of particles at all but of vibrations of energy. The rishis and maharishis who first formulated ayurveda acknowledged this from their own findings, based on the study of the human nervous system. Meditating at a highly refined level, they discerned these energetic vibrations, which together made up the primordial humming sound, Om. Thus the use of a mantra was discovered to harness the power of harmonious vibrations.

There are various sounds that can be used as mantras. Being a meaningless sound, the mantra does not keep the mind on the surface in the way that contemplation, visualization or concentration techniques do. It allows it instead to be active yet undirected, free to settle toward a deep silence.

The best way to learn to meditate is with a teacher trained in transcendental meditation who will choose the appropriate mantra for you and show you how to use it. The course generally consists of a number of sessions, interspersed with your own practice at home, so you can check your progress and discuss any difficulties.

When you meditate at home, try to do it at the same time and place each day. It is short, regular practice that builds the benefits, rather than the occasional long session. Start with one, or preferably two, ten-minute daily sessions, one in the morning, the other in the evening before you have eaten and not after you have drunk alcohol. If you are very tired you will probably fall asleep until the meditation clears the fatigue. Take the phone off the hook or switch on the answering machine and do whatever else is necessary to avoid being disturbed. Find a quiet spot, wear loose, comfortable clothing and take off your shoes. When you become adept, though, you will be able to meditate at any time and in all kinds of places, even when there is noise or other people are around.

If you find it comfortable, you can sit cross-legged on the floor—and if you're super-flexible and

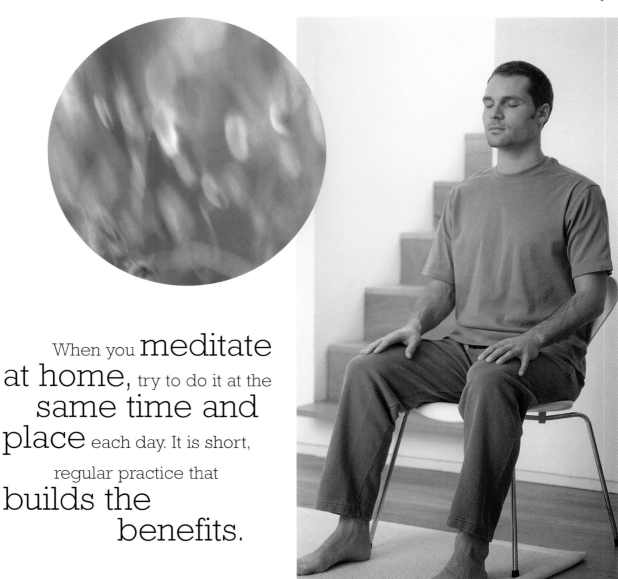

When you **meditate at home,** try to do it at the **same time and place** each day. It is short, regular practice that **builds the benefits.**

it is not an effort to sustain, you can even do a more complicated position like a lotus or half-lotus, though this does not affect the quality of your meditation. It is important for you to be comfortable in the position you choose for the entire length of your meditation, although moving and fidgeting is allowed! Sit reasonably upright, and if you know your back will ache after five minutes, lean against a piece of furniture or sit in a straight-backed chair with your feet flat on the floor.

Before you begin, take a few moments to focus on your body. Take some slow, deep breaths and try to let go of any areas of tension. Common ones are the shoulders and back, but many people hold tension, without realizing it, all over their bodies, as well as in the face and scalp. Finally, scan your mind for immediate thoughts and worries. Observe them and set them aside to deal with later. Now let the mantra come into your mind and begin your meditation.

Breathing techniques

There are various ways in which the breath can be used to relax the body and mind and increase awareness. Breathing techniques are particularly useful in treating insomnia. They are beneficial, too, as a means of stress relief throughout the day.

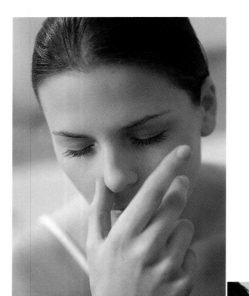

◀ Pranayama
This is simply alternate breathing—you use one nostril at a time. This slows down the breath and creates a feeling of calm.

1 Sit on a chair that supports your spine so that you feel comfortable and relaxed. If you prefer, you can kneel or sit cross-legged on the floor, but your back must be as straight as possible and held without tension. Choose whichever position is most comfortable for you—this will support your pranayama best.

2 Close your eyes and breathe in. With your left hand resting in your lap, lift your right hand up to be on a level with your face and, using your thumb, close your right nostril.

3 Exhale through your left nostril, slowly and easily. Then breathe in, slowly and easily again.

4 Now close off your left nostril with the middle finger of your right hand. Exhale, then inhale slowly through the right nostril.

5 Continue, alternating nostrils, for about five minutes. Your breathing should be as natural as possible, not exaggerated, though it may be a little slower and deeper than usual.

6 After five minutes, sit quietly with your eyes closed and breathe normally for a

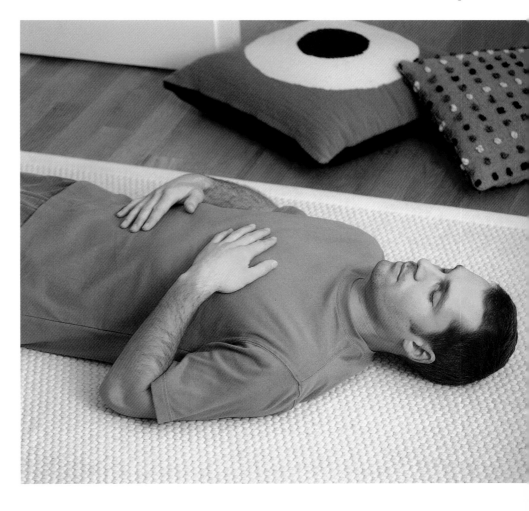

Abdominal breathing ▶

1 Lie in the corpse pose (see page 107) on a blanket on the floor, covering yourself with another blanket if you feel cold. Your spine should be in one long line, continuing up through the neck to the top of the head. Let your feet and legs roll out so they are relaxed and place your arms a little way from your sides, palms facing upwards. Check your body for signs of tension and release as much as you can.

2 Place one hand on your abdomen and the other on your chest. Feel your body move with your breath. If the hand on your chest moves more than the one on your abdomen, your breath is only reaching a small proportion of your body.

3 On the next breath, exhale as fully as you can so that you push the air out from the bottom of your lungs. Now breathe in through your nose again for as long as you can until you feel your abdomen rise, not just your chest.

4 Inhaling and exhaling only through the nose, continue to take long, slow abdominal breaths for a few minutes.

5 Return to your normal breathing for a few minutes before getting up.

Case history

A very successful and dynamic businesswoman (vata/pitta) in her mid-thirties found that the Pitta side of her makeup would escalate in the late mornings (pitta time) and she was in danger of literally losing her cool. She would disappear from the office and slip to the bathroom to practice her pranayama for a few minutes. This left her feeling relaxed and calm. The only problem was that her colleagues noticed the dramatic change and her radiant calm and assumed she had a bowel problem!

Chapter seven

The treatment spa

It is now possible to find professional treatments available from therapists trained in European ayurveda. Traditional ayurveda has treatments that most Westerners would find unpalatable – such as emesis (induced vomiting), blood-letting, purges and enemas. Unlike traditional ayurveda, however, European ayurveda spas do not seek to function as medical centers or hospitals providing treatment for specific diseases. Nevertheless, by profoundly detoxifying and relaxing both mind and body, they remove many of the risk factors associated with serious conditions, as well as relieving stress-related problems. They also provide a deeply relaxing and rejuvenating break for anyone with a high-stress life. A very light diet is usually given during your stay at the spa as these treatments are deeply purifying and the body is focussed on the elimination of toxins. Rest and relaxation are encouraged and you take only the gentlest of exercise – such as walking and yoga. Most people find they sleep more deeply than they have for years, especially if they have been under stress, and leave feeling refreshed and relaxed.

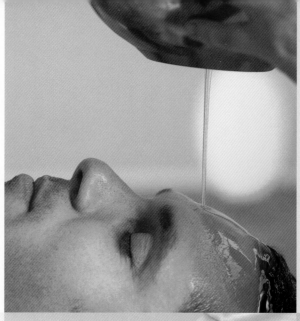

Vata people

Massage: warm sesame oil on the body and coconut oil on the head in hot weather and sunflower or olive oil in cold weather

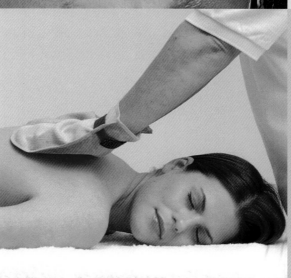

Pitta people

Massage: sesame oil or coconut oil if it is too warm

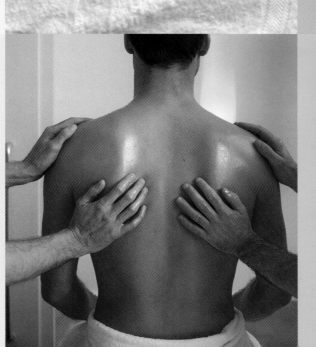

Kapha people

Massage: firm deep massage with bare hands or raw silk gloves

Therapeutic massage

Ayurvedic massage is quite different from the forms better known in the West. All of the massages are performed, in silence, by two therapists working in unison. The strokes used are quite different than Western ones—and vary, too, according to your dosha. The treatments generally last longer and the oil used is both individually created for your dosha and applied hot. Heat is a purifying factor in ayurvedic massage. All of these elements result in a treatment that is profoundly relaxing, therapeutic and detoxifying.

Rejuvenating massage

According to the ancient Indian texts, a course of these therapeutic massages, combined with a purifying ayurvedic diet, "renews bodily tissues and strengthens the senses, thus preventing aging and giving 100 years of life." This may seem a rather extravagant claim, but research has shown that ayurvedic treatment can have remarkable effects. A week in an ayurvedic spa has been seen to dispel accumulated toxins and reduce anxiety, fatigue and cardiovascular risk factors, including cholesterol levels, and (according to the Morgan Test, which measures biological age) your physiological age by, on average, a little under five years.

When you go to an ayurvedic spa, one of the first things likely to strike you is how calm and quiet it is. There is no background music and treatments take place in silence, except for the occasional request to turn over. You are completely naked during the massage and, while towels are used to cover the parts not being massaged, they are often quite small! However, although you may feel unusually exposed from time to time, you never feel cold and one of the first things you notice in an ayurvedic

treatment room is how warm it is. Any feelings of embarrassment tend to disappear within minutes—massages are deeply relaxing and they are always given by therapists who are the same sex as you.

Case history

HRH the Prince Andrew, Duke of York, has been a devotee of European ayurveda for the last five years. He has a four-day full panchakarma once a year and, being Pitta/Kapha, he has the treatment in the winter months, usually after Christmas. He then follows the three-day program with a fluid day in the summer. The jibes about his weight are now a thing of the past and he both looks and feels healthier, happier and more vibrant.

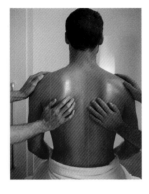

Abhyanga

The most widely used body massage is Abhyanga—translated as "loving hands." This is a very soothing, gentle massage and is designed to stimulate the release of toxins from the cells and circulation to the subcutaneous tissues. There are three types—vata, pitta and kapha—which vary both in depth and speed of stroke and in length—between thirty five minutes and an hour.

The massage begins while you are seated in a chair, still wrapped in a robe. Your feet are carefully washed, dried and placed on a hot-water bottle. Your shoulders, face and head—including even your ears—are massaged with warm oil. The oil is generally sesame, as this has its own therapeutic properties (see page 134), but those with highly sensitive skin may need a less robust oil. This base oil is often scented with other therapeutic oils, created to suit your dosha or imbalance. This preliminary seated massage is repeated at the beginning of all the massage treatments below. After this initial seated massage, you are led to the treatment table, where your back and arms are massaged while you sit at the edge of the table, and then you lie down for a long body massage with the two therapists working in complete synchronicity. Most people find that because there are four hands rather than two they do not focus on one particular area and drift instead into a state of deep relaxation. And as the oil is hot, muscles relax much more quickly and profoundly. At the end of this massage you are wrapped in warm towels and left to rest for about twenty minutes.

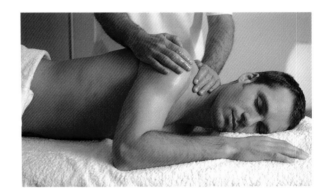

Shirodhara

Abhyanga is often combined with Shirodhara, which does for the mind what the first massage has done for the body. It is particularly settling for vata disorders, such as insomnia and anxiety, and it profoundly relaxes the central nervous system. Lying on your back with your head tipped gently back, a thin drizzle of sesame oil passes slowly back and forth across your brow, like a pendulum, pausing almost imperceptibly each time it reaches the center or the temples. It lasts for twenty minutes and many people compare its effects to transcendence, the meditator's state of bliss. After Shirodhara, you rest in bed for around an hour—either in a completely relaxed state or, after a few minutes, fast asleep.

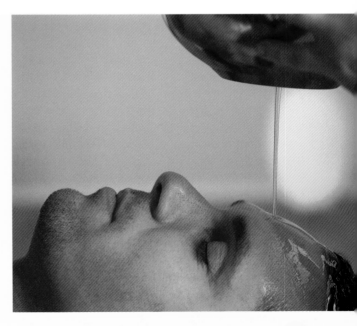

131

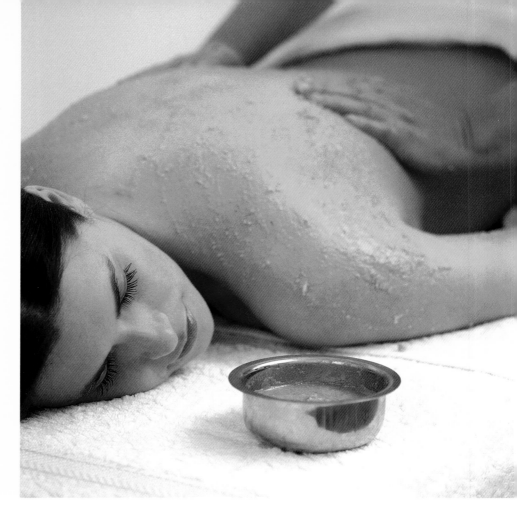

Urdvatana

This very invigorating massage is one that uses a specially blended herbal paste, made with various grains, flours, herbs and oils. It cleanses, exfoliates, tones and tightens the skin, leaving it feeling fresh, young and silky-smooth. It increases circulation, promotes weight loss and is very effective for cellulite.

Vishesh

This massage is particularly suitable for Kaphas. It involves firm, squeezing movements and is generally preferred by people who have a large, strong physique and enjoy a massage that gives a deeper pressure. It is designed to remove deep-rooted toxins from the physiology.

Pinda abhyanga

This is a nourishing massage that requires three people, rather than the usual two, because one is busy boiling up the boluses—muslin bags full of rice, cooked in herbalized milk—with which you are massaged. The smell is unmistakable and it is rather like being massaged with rice pudding. It transforms dry, rough skin into a soft, silky, smooth texture with a satin gleam. You need a long shower afterwards to get rid of the starchy residue, but it has a profoundly relaxing and soothing effect.

Pizzichilli

This was known in India as the "royal treatment" and was reserved for the maharajahs. It is very heating and relaxing and beloved by Vatas in particular, for whom it is very balancing and soothing —Pittas can find it makes them uncomfortably hot. Gallons of warm oil are poured over you while two therapists gently massage the oil into your body. As it penetrates the skin, it releases deep-seated aches and pains and brings flexibility to your joints.

Swedana

This is an ayurvedic version of a steam bath. It softens and dilates the channels of the body, allowing the impurities to move out of fatty tissues for elimination and is particularly balancing for Vata and Kapha types. It is generally given at the end of another massage. You are left to rest after the first massage for ten minutes and then a specially designed tent is placed over your body, leaving your face and head clear. The tent is then filled with a continuous flow of herbalized steam which surrounds your body, the therapists keeping your face and head cool with applications of coconut oil and cool water-filled towels.

Netra tarpana

This is an eye treatment which is soothing and relaxing and particularly beneficial for anyone suffering ill-effects from computers, pollution or whose eyes feel strained. The eyes are a pitta organ, the secondary seat of pitta, and they should never get hot. This cools not only the eyes but the mind. First you have a facial massage, then hot towels are wrapped gently around your face. Dough rings are placed around your eyes and filled with special cooling oils or ghee to soothe and bathe them. It can be quite scary to open your eyes but, when you do, your vision is bathed in a golden glow and you do some simple eye exercises to help the ghee take effect. This sounds like a very strange process but it does have a deeply relaxing effect and it certainly makes you realize how much tension is stored in the eyes.

Kati basti

An external, localized massage using heat and specific herbalized oils on the lower back, particularly designed for anyone who suffers from lower back pain. It eases rigidity of the lower spine and strengthens the bone tissue in that area.

Marma therapy

This is not widely available and must only ever be given by a qualified practitioner, as it is a very powerful treatment. In ayurveda, a marma point is a crucial meeting point of the flesh, veins, arteries, tendons, bones and joints. Marma points are similar to, though not the same as, the meridian points of Chinese acupuncture. While marma points are stimulated gently during other European ayurvedic massages, in marma therapy they are the focus of the treatment. This is the only massage in European ayurveda to be administered by one therapist and it can be greatly enhanced by using specific essential oils on particular marma points. It is especially effective for soothing vata's imbalances and emotional blockages.

Garshan

This massage has a similar effect to Urdvatana, increasing circulation, promoting weight loss and reducing cellulite by clearing away impurities that may be blocking the system. The therapists wear raw silk gloves and give a brisk, enlivening massage, creating friction and static electricity on the surface of the skin. You can also buy the gloves to use at home.

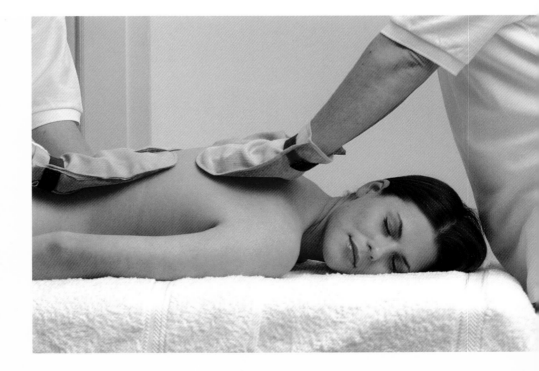

Self-massage

As the benefits of massage are so wide-ranging, European ayurveda recommends that you give yourself a daily massage. The best time to do this is in the morning before you take a bath or shower. You need just a few minutes for the massage if you are in a hurry, though the longer you massage and keep the oil on before washing, the better. So if you are not going out, you could leave it to absorb for several hours. This is particularly true for the oil on your scalp. However, it is better to give yourself a quick two-minute massage in the morning rather than none at all. As it is so settling and sooth-ing, you can also give yourself a foot massage if you have trouble sleeping at night. In this case, though, it is probably a good idea to wear thin cotton socks to sleep in to prevent the oil from staining the sheets.

Sesame oil

The best oil for your massage is sesame oil. If you react badly to sesame oil—if, for instance, it gives you a rash—you can use sunflower oil. Pitta types may find it too heating, particularly in the summer, in which case cooling coconut oil will be more suitable.

According to European ayurveda, sesame oil is, however, regarded as the most beneficial oil to use, because it is so settling and nourishing for the body. It is believed to purify the digestive system, lubricate the joints and muscles, remove ama (toxins) from the system and rejuvenate the tissues—and so delay the signs of aging and ensure a strong and healthy old age. Oil naturally lubricates and softens the skin. Because sesame oil contains antioxidants that fight the free radicals which are the first cause of so many degenerative diseases, it is thought to enhance the immune system. The act of massage itself is very calming to the mind and emotions.

For the best results, use cold-pressed oil and "ripen" before use—this entails heating to 212°F. Place two teacups of oil in a saucepan and add one or two drops of water. Heat slowly and watch the

oil all the time—oil is inflammable, so never leave the room while it is heating up. As the oil warms up, it makes a crackling sound, which is the water boil-ing off. When the crackling has stopped, the oil has reached the correct temperature. Allow the oil to cool and store in a bottle. If you have not used up all the oil within one month, it will need to be ripened again. Never refrigerate the oil.

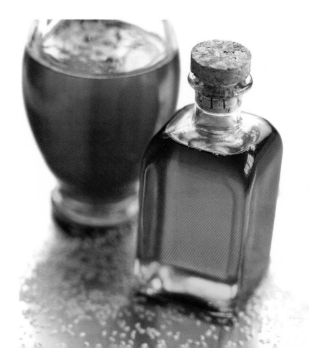

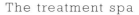

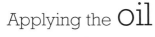

Applying the Oil

1 Put some towels on the floor of a warm room where you are going to give yourself the massage. Warm a quarter of a teacup of oil to just above body temperature by placing it in a container of hot water or on top of a radiator. Apply the oil all over the body, including the scalp, the hair and the soles of the feet.

2 Begin the massage with the head. Circle the scalp with vigorous movements, then move to the outer ears and face, massaging these more gently. Massage the neck and as much as you can of the back. Around the joints, use a circular motion; for longer sections use a straight, sweeping movement.

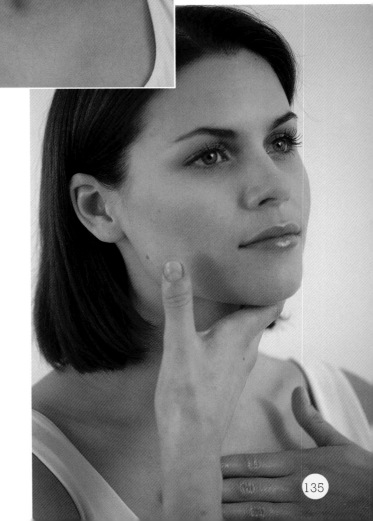

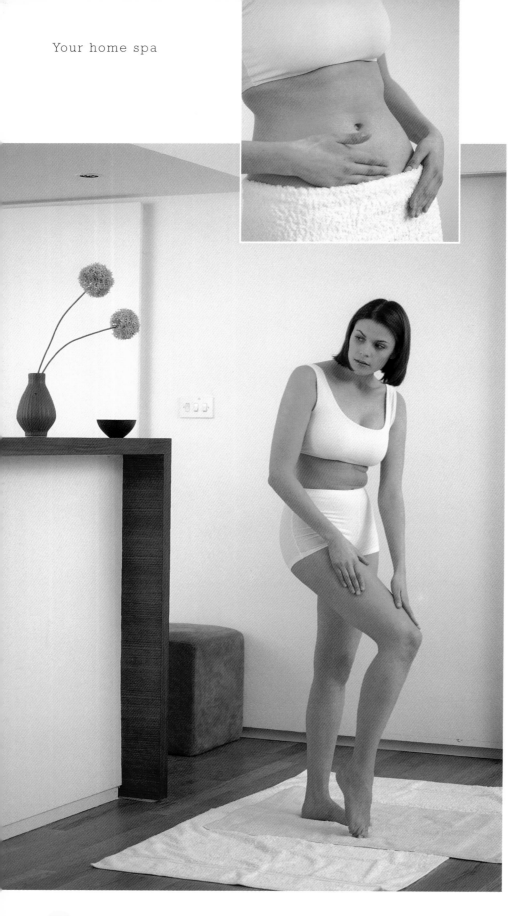

3 Next, massage the arms, the chest and the stomach, using a gentle clockwise movement over the abdomen.

4 Massage the legs vigorously with long, sweeping strokes, except for the ankles, knees and hips, where you should use a circular movement again.

5 Finally, massage the feet, paying particular attention to the soles.

6 Now is a good time to have breakfast, do your yoga and any other part of your routine—except for meditation or breathing techniques—while the oil absorbs. Always have a bath or shower before you meditate.

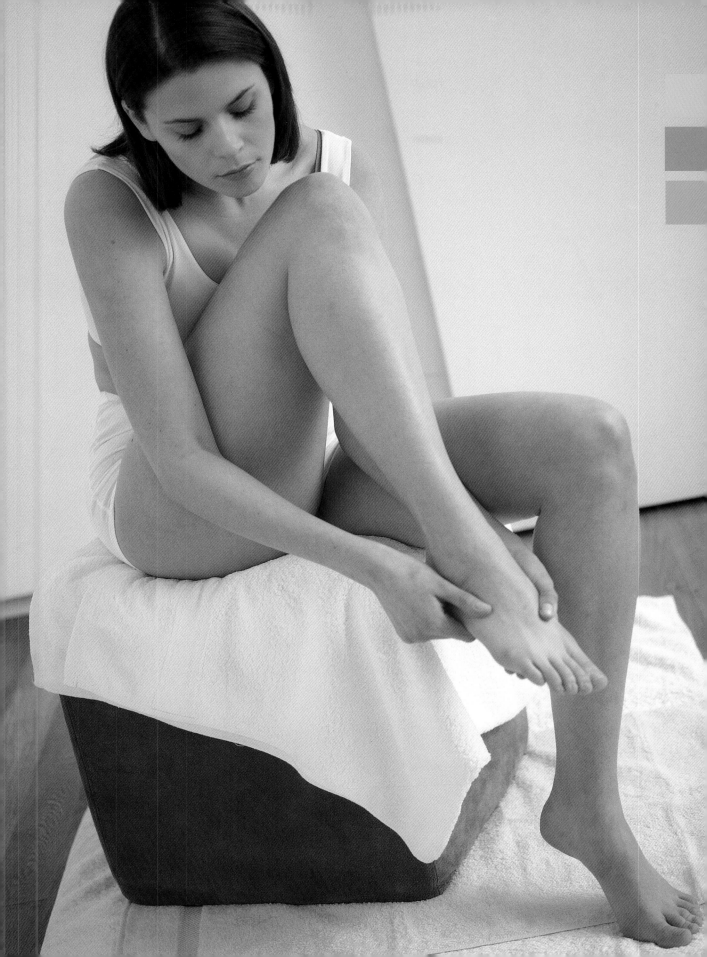

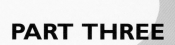

PART THREE

Ayurveda throughout your life

While diet, exercise and meditation are the fundamental ayurvedic tools for achieving a state of health and balance within ourselves, ayurvedic principles extend throughout every activity, situation and relationship in our lives. This means that we can look beyond ourselves and, seeing the world through ayurvedic eyes, create a sense of harmony in our living and working environments, with family, friends and colleagues and in all our activities. Once you know the conditions, situations or activities that are likely to aggravate your particular dosha or put you out of balance, you can take steps to avoid them or to counteract their effects.

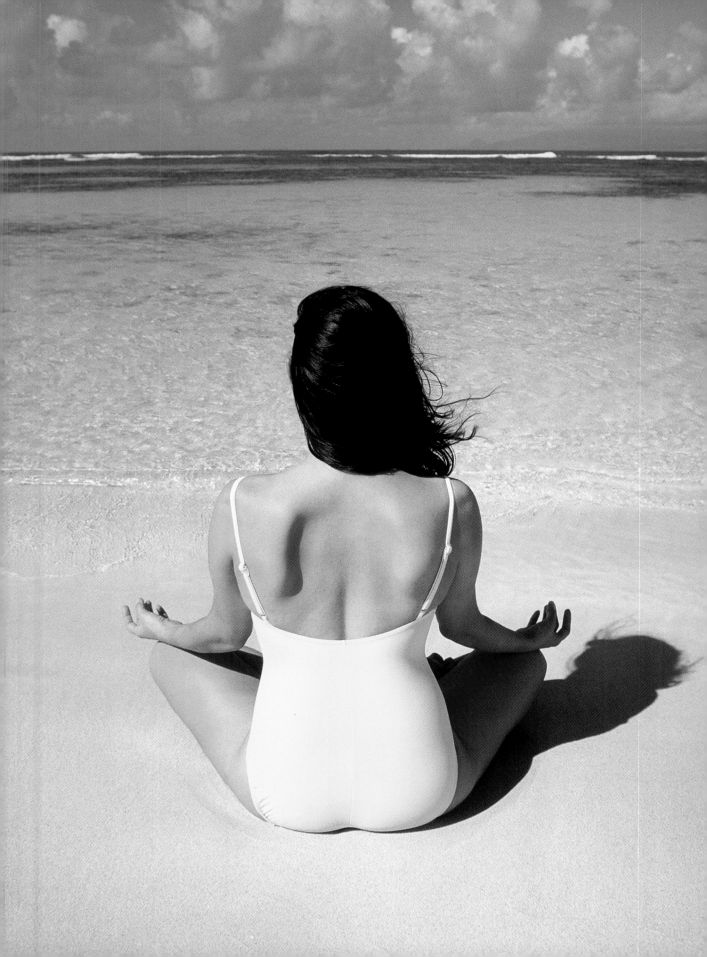

Chapter eight

Creating your perfect environment

Everyone knows that sense of walking into a room and feeling instantly at home. There is something in the atmosphere that seems to make it just right for you. However, the different doshic types will respond in this way to very different environments and need to create very specific interiors to feel relaxed and in harmony with their homes. The same is true of gardens and outdoor environments, with each dosha feeling comfortable in a different kind of space. The importance of creating the right kind of living space for yourself cannot be exaggerated. Everyone needs to be able to come home and feel a moment of pleasure as they step through the door. Ayurveda encourages a clean, tidy, light living space, enhanced by colors that balance your doshic makeup, and pleasant sounds and scents. If you share your home with a partner, children or friends, there will inevitably be more than one doshic type in the house. In this case, you need to aim for a tri-doshic approach that will create a harmonious environment for everyone. Go for creams and magnolias—not white— in shared rooms, and then bedrooms and studies can be painted in the color appropriate for each individual.

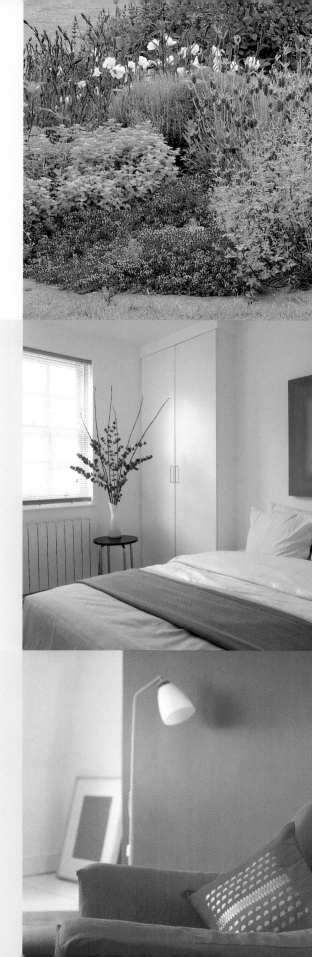

Vata people

Home:
natural fibers and fabrics, big windows, rounded shapes

Garden:
pastel flowers, cottage garden

Career:
actor, dancer, artist, writer, designer

Pitta people

Home
angular shapes, uncluttered, formal style—Georgian or modern

Garden:
water features, formal garden, pale-colored flowers

Career:
manager, lawyer, politician, surgeon, chef, comedian

Kapha people

Home
comfortable, cozy, warm colors

Garden:
sun-trap, bold, colorful flowers

Career:
nurse, administrator, gardener, counsellor

Vata home & garden

Vatas are always on the move, either physically or mentally, and, with comparatively low reserves of energy, have a tendency to get stressed and tired. So Vatas' homes need to be a haven of peace and comfort—a place to wind down, recuperate and relax.

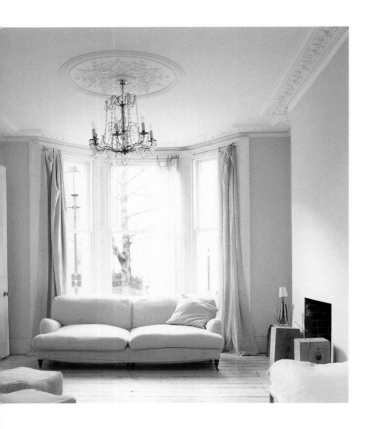

Natural comfort

The key word in a Vata person's home is "natural." You should choose natural fibers and fabrics for furniture and other furnishings—ideal Vata window dressings, for instance, would be wooden or bamboo, and rice-paper blinds, cotton or linen curtains. Upholstery, carpets and cushions should be in natural fabrics, too, or you could throw wool,

silk or cotton rugs on top of wooden floors. The same natural look goes for colors. Over-bright, artificial-looking or fluorescent colors simply upset Vatas. You prefer warm pastel colors and light blues and greens—go for a light, bright overall look.

Light is, in fact, very important to Vatas. You like big windows and airy, spacious rooms and a feeling of openness in your home. Although you take pleasure in well-crafted objects, paintings and decorative touches—and you will give a lot of thought to getting these just right—you shouldn't have too many of them. Clutter upsets and un-settles Vatas.

While you like a room to have a feeling of spaciousness to it, it should be warm, comfortable and, above all, draft-free. You cannot relax in a cold, drafty house, nor in one that has too many angles and sharp corners. Vatas love to have archways opening one room into another and arranging furniture into pleasing, not too regular, patterns. Choose furniture that has soft rounded shapes—circular tables, sofas with round arms, oval or circular mirrors.

Vatas enjoy having plants and flowers inside the house, particularly ones with sweet smells and delicate colors and shapes, such as roses and sweet peas. You are soothed by silence or gentle sounds, such as quiet, classical music or the occasional sound of a wooden wind chime.

Your favorite style is the cottage garden ...
full of old-fashioned, sweet-smelling pastel flowers.

Vatas' garden

The ideal outside space for Vatas is, like your home, a warm, secure haven. A walled garden protecting you from wind and drafts, with a sunny spot for basking, is perfect. Your favorite style is the cottage garden, full of archways, irregularly shaped flowerbeds and old-fashioned, sweet-smelling pastel flowers like roses, sweet peas, lilies, hollyhocks, lavender, pinks, lily-of-the-valley, hyacinths and delphiniums.

Vatas love the sound of nature, too, especially that of leaves rustled by the breeze. An ideal garden feature for a Vata is a pagoda or some other form of seating with a big-leafed vine or climber growing around it, giving both shelter and a pleasing, natural sound. If you have a lot of space or you are able to garden on an ambitious scale, the Vata person's ultimate garden feature would be a maze, full of hidden corners, irregular shapes and surprising treasures to find along the way—a

statue here, a fountain there. The paths should always be gently winding with no sharp corners and preferably grassy. Vatas' gardens should have some grass, because airy Vatas always need to be grounded and walking barefoot on the grass is one of the best ways of achieving this.

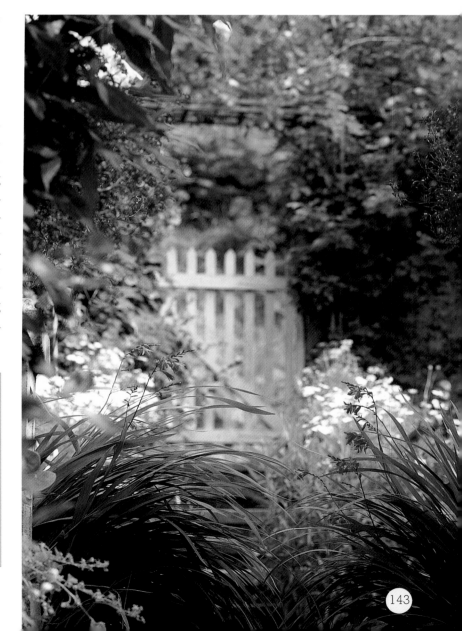

vata chooses

- Rounded shapes
- Comfortable and draft-free environments
- Warm pastel colors and light blues and greens
- Natural fibers, fabrics
- Sweet-smelling flowers

Pitta home & garden

Pitta's fiery personality needs a home that will cool and soothe it into a mellow mood. You like order and formality in both home and garden, and tend to go for boardroom sumptuousness or minimalist chic.

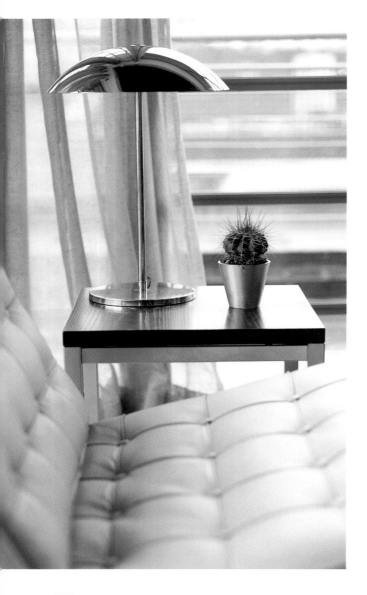

Pitta precision

Pittas hate clutter and strive toward neatness and straight lines—pictures must be precisely aligned, rugs straight and unrumpled, and furniture set at the correct angles. Pittas are very fond of angles and favor square furniture, such as dining tables and chairs. You like a highly polished, formal look—the symmetrical beauty of Georgian furniture and architecture is your favorite. For the same reason, you love dado rails that split a wall into neat sections, especially if one is covered in neat, narrowly striped wallpaper. You particularly like big desks, especially ones with a leather top, which symbolize quality and authority.

If you are not a traditionalist, you are likely to be an absolute modernist with everything pared down to the utmost minimalism. For this look, you like chrome and leather furniture—you love leather not only because of its quality but also because of its smell—and low, angled tables and a few well-chosen modern objects. That's enough.

Whichever of these two extremes you choose, color is vital if all that Pitta precision is not to become too overpowering. Soothe your environment with cooling blues and lilacs—and this will create a cooling, pacifying atmosphere. You are very fond of pictures and the most balancing for your dosha are landscapes, especially seascapes or waterfalls—water in any form is very soothing for Pitta types. Best of all is a big window with a view straight out to sea!

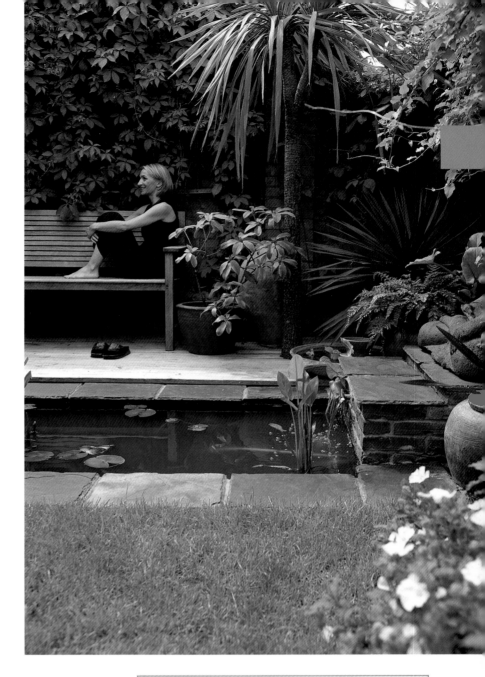

A formal garden

Water is the most important feature in Pittas' gardens: a pond, a fountain, a splash pool, a waterfall or a swimming pool. Depending on the size of your garden, the more water that can be fitted into it the better. Pittas find it very relaxing to sit and look at water, so put a seat or a patch of grass next to it where you can spend some time in quiet reflection. Above all, make sure you will be sitting in a shady spot. If you are in full sun, all that heat will undermine the balancing and soothing effects of the water. If you have room for a pond, many water plants will enhance the cooling effect. Try the pure white calla lily (*Calla palustris*), blue water iris, water lilies and plenty of stately water grasses.

You will almost certainly prefer a formal garden with flowers in rows and well-defined beds. Soften this with color—go for pale blues, lavenders and creams—and scents. Again, the scents should be cooling, so choose plants such as lavender, *nicotiana* (tobacco plant), coniferous trees and shrubs and a whole host of herbs—mint, sage, thyme—in a carefully laid-out knot garden.

pitta chooses

- Straight lines and angular shapes
- Cooling colors
- Highly polished formal look
- Gardens with water features

Depending on the size of your garden, the more water that can be fitted into it the better.

Kapha home & garden

Kaphas love comfort and are likely to have the most cozy home of any dosha. Too much comfort, though, and you will find your home fails to offer you the stimulation you need. For the perfect environment, think bold and bright.

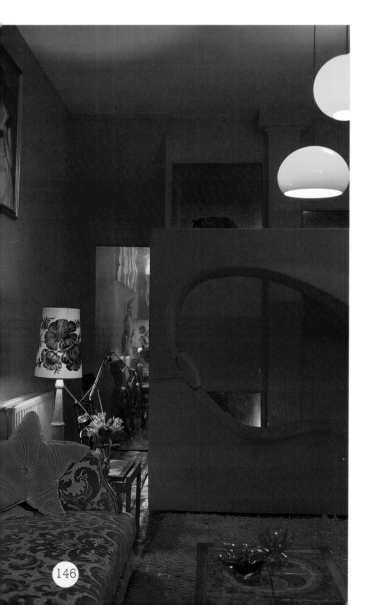

Kapha chooses

- Big, comfy furniture
- Bright lights, and even moving lights
- Lots of personal mementoes and knick-knacks
- Bold colors in vibrant shades
- A sun-trap in the garden

Cozy Kapha

Kaphas will always go for comfort. Your living room will be filled with big, comfy sofas, covered in squashy cushions. You'll have a footstool or a chair that gives you a back massage while you watch television and a big table that you can reach without having to stretch for food, drink and the remote control!

Kaphas love to feel secure and, besides having giant-sized, comfortable furniture, also tend to accumulate lots of mementoes and collections. Every shelf and surface is likely to have an array of knick-knacks, gifts from friends, holiday souvenirs or little collections of objects that appeal—from beach pebbles to fine china. These collections can look great if you keep them under control and you can feel quite forlorn without them. But don't let them take over the room—it's good to see the table top now and again!

The great potential danger in the Kapha person's home is for it to get too cozy and comfortable and for you to never make any changes or updates. The result of this is that you start to feel bored and listless and your home stops being the stimulating environment you need. One of the most effective ways to achieve the interior that will best suit you is to use plenty of color. Kaphas need bold, bright colors and you are the only one of the three doshas who can live with reds and oranges and really strong, vibrant shades. Experiment with small splashes of brightness on cushions, rugs, curtains and pictures—or even paint the whole room an intense color.

Kaphas don't mind small rooms—these add to their sense of security. You do need light, but, unlike the case with Vatas and Pittas, this can be just as effective from an artificial source. In particular, the stimulus of moving light is beneficial—a lava lamp is an ideal present for Kaphas, and they do love twinkly Christmas trees! For the rest of the year, go for very bright lights—the shinier the better.

Color crazy

Kaphas' gardens should be full of color. Forget Pittas' cooling blues and Vatas' pastel prettiness—what you need is a positive riot of color. Grow deep flowerbeds with all the big, bold flowers you can think of—in the brightest yellows, reds and oranges. Ideal Kapha plants include deep red peonies, marigolds, tulips, sunflowers, geraniums, Busy Lizzies, hollyhocks, red hot pokers (*Kniphofia*), poppies, asters, chrysanthemums and tiger lilies. Shapes, too, can be bold and architectural—with spiky grasses and palms. Cover paths in crunchy-sounding pebbles and put up a greenhouse so you can appreciate its steamy heat. Ideally, your garden should be a sun-trap. Best of all is a garden with a red-brick wall that can be covered in honeysuckle or big-flowered clematis—an ideal place to bask in the heat.

Kaphas need **bold, bright** colors and you are the only one of the three doshas who can live with **reds and oranges** and really strong, vibrant shades.

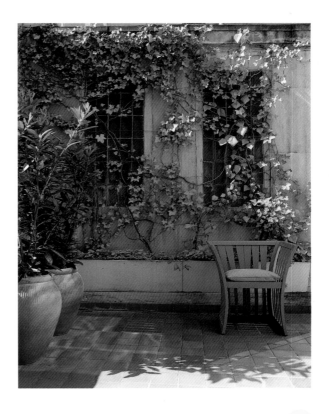

Work

The sort of work that you do and the workplace that you do it in can either antagonize or calm your leading dosha or imbalance. Each type is drawn naturally to certain kinds of work and this tends to increase the dominant dosha. Pittas, for instance, love food and pitta is the most common principal dosha for a chef. The heat of the kitchen, however, inflames Pitta—leading to the caricature of the fiery-tempered prima donna!

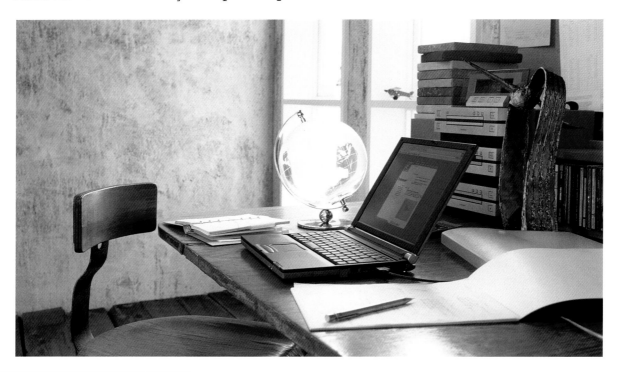

Case history

Pacifying a Pitta Imbalance
The sea has a uniquely calming effect on Pittas. One highly successful businessman in his late forties, a regular visitor to the European Ayurveda spa, was a Pitta type. Because he was under great stress, with constant pressure and demands, he would often find himself reaching boiling point. When it got really bad he was advised to take himself out of the city and drive to the nearest point on the coast. He then spent a couple of hours walking by the sea, until he felt cooled and calmed, able to see things in perspective once more. On later visits to the spa, he confirmed that the technique had not only worked, but probably also saved his sanity.

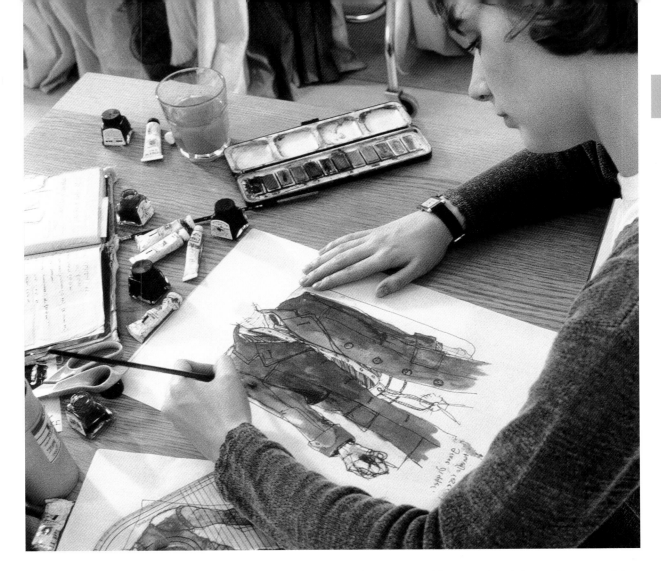

Vatas at work

Vatas have great enthusiasm, inventiveness and creative ability. You are drawn to work that has an artistic element—many dancers, actors, artists, writers and designers are strongly Vata. It is vital for you to express your creativity—if not at work, you need to find another outlet for it—but this should be balanced with grounding activity and you should beware of wearing yourself out in nervous exhaustion. Try to pace yourself so that your initial enthusiasm for a new project does not use up all your energy reserves and you can see it through to its end.

Being so imaginative, your ideas tend to come thick and fast, but this means you are also likely to change your mind often. One priority at a time should be tackled: think it through thoroughly and stick to your decisions. Whenever possible, delegate repetitive, routine jobs and practicalities to others who cope better with them and, above all, take steps to avoid and reduce stress—Vatas suffer more from stress and stress-related problems than the other two doshas.

Many working environments tend to increase vata. Working in front of a computer screen all day (take plenty of breaks away from the desk), talking on the phone, travel of any kind (but especially air travel) and air-conditioned shops and offices all aggravate vata and leave you feeling anxious or exhausted.

Cold, drafty workplaces also increase vata, as does working too close to an open door or window, and high noise levels are similarly disturbing to Vatas. The ideal workplace has plenty of space and natural light, is quiet, warm and painted in a soft pastel color.

Pittas at work

In balance, Pittas are clear-sighted, ambitious and goal-oriented. You admire authority and have a great love of order, and are often natural leaders in the workplace. You have supreme confidence, an excellent memory and enjoy a challenge, and all of this makes you an asset in any business. You excel in particular in management, the law, politics (where you have a strong will to win!) and the financial sector and, because of your precision and attention to detail, you would also make a good surgeon. Because of your love of food, you are often drawn to the idea of cooking for a living and, with your razor-sharp wit and excellent timing, you could make a very successful stand-up comedian.

Out of balance, however, you can become aggressive and difficult with colleagues, prone to conflict and often blaming others if you encounter a problem. You do not respond well to criticism—in fact, you tend to react to it with hostility—and, while your decisive mind leads you to hold strong opinions that you defend keenly, you should try to listen more calmly to the viewpoints of others.

You never shy away from a challenge—and will usually handle one very well—but try to keep things in perspective and don't allow yourself to become over-competitive as this will increase pitta and tend to make you more likely to find yourself in conflict with others. You love the challenge of business and are the likeliest of the doshas to become a workaholic—it is vital to balance your tremendous drive and determination with a calming environment and activities. Otherwise, beware! He may be a comic creation, but Basil in

Fawlty Towers is a dangerously accurate portrayal of the temperament of someone with an extreme pitta imbalance.

Excessive use of computers—with the inevitable focus and concentration on a small screen—will greatly aggravate Pittas. Take regular breaks and use a pacifying aroma oil, such as lavender, in the office if you are sitting at a desk for much of the day. Try to sit by a window that you can open in hot weather and have a fan on your desk to keep you cool in every sense. An overheated workplace will inflame pitta. It is vital that you eat a good lunch every day, as hunger dangerously aggravates pitta, and you should put off making important decisions or holding key meetings until you have had your lunch. Because you are such a perfectionist, you work best in an environment that is relaxing and helps prevent you from pushing yourself too hard. Working with a small group of friends—people who know you well enough to give you a wide berth when you are at your most Pitta!—would be the most supportive situation for you.

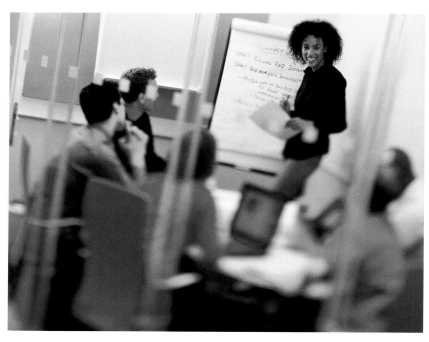

Kaphas at work

Kaphas are calm and stable, with lots of patience, strength and an inbuilt desire to help others. You make a terrific nurse or counsellor and excel in any job that entails caring for other people. You also have great reserves of physical strength, endurance and energy, and are the most able of any of the doshas to do tasking, manual work—while your natural affinity with the earth means you make a good builder or farmer. With an excellent memory, good planning skills and the ability to see projects through from beginning to end, you are a very good administrator and long-term planner. You are also the safest driver (see pages 152–3) and machine operator and the least likely to have accidents with vehicles or mechanical equipment.

Naturally conservative, Kaphas tend not to rock the boat and fit well into large companies, where you tend to have lots of friends, as you are so kind and considerate to others. You enjoy the sense of security this brings—unlike the other doshas, it is hard for you to break away and change your job or career—but you should take care that you do not become too set in your ways. You have a tendency to resist change of any kind because you are so keen to support the status quo. Lack of growth and stimulus results in an excess of kapha, however, and this slows you down, leaving you feeling dull and bored. At its most extreme, excess kapha leads to a head-in-the-sand approach to life—you hope that if you ignore a challenge, it will go away.

In fact, Kaphas need the stimulation of challenge at work, both mentally and physically. Although you are reluctant to do it because you hate to be away from home and family, travel can be a beneficial part of your work. You do not mind routine or even monotony in your job, but if you don't find stimulation at work, it is vital that you find it else-where—becoming a chess champion in your spare time, for instance.

Like Vatas, Kaphas need a warm, dry environment if you are to work indoors, though you are

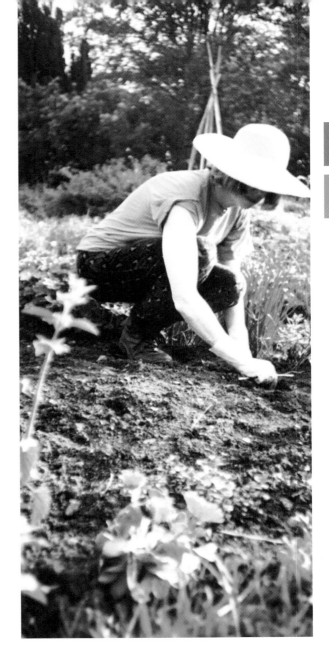

You have great reserves of

physical strength,

endurance and energy.

ideally suited, too, to working outside. If you don't have a job that requires any physical activity, it is important that you take very regular, preferably daily, exercise, or you will start to feel lethargic and bored. Give yourself challenges at work and don't back down and become self-effacing at the thought of promotion—be bold!

Vacations and travel

Nowhere is it so immediately obvious that each dosha is fundamentally different than when it comes to how they spend their vacations.

Vatas love warmth and sun and, despite the tendency to like constant movement and change for its own sake, you are best suited to staying in one beautiful, relaxing spot and just soaking up the atmosphere. Vacations in cold climates and especially at high altitudes are not good for Vatas—you need to be as grounded as possible. With a predominantly Vata prakriti myself, I know the place I felt most instantly relaxed was on the banks of the Dead Sea in Jordan—the lowest point on earth and, of course, very hot and dry.

Kaphas may want to join Vatas and lie in the sun all day but, in fact, you are better off with a more stimulating activity-based holiday—the more physical the better. You do need the sun, though, and most importantly a dry climate—humidity will aggravate Kaphas. Pittas, on the other hand, are top skiers, surfers and hang-gliders. You need a cooling climate and a challenge and should avoid a hot climate at all costs.

Doshas in the car

The three doshas have very definite characteristics when it comes to driving and, it has to be said, if I ever had a chauffeur, I'd choose a Kapha every time. Kaphas are slow but safe—you stick to the speed limit and never feel intimidated into driving faster than you feel is right. You may infuriate other

Flight routine

All forms of travel increase vata, whatever your dominant dosha, and flying aggravates it most of all. Long-haul flights are particularly trying, whatever your prakriti, because crossing time zones is a far from natural experience. Jet-lag can be minimized and recovery from it speeded up with the following routine:

■ On the morning of departure, have a self-massage, Sun Salutation routine, followed by a warm bath with five to ten drops of lavender oil. Rub a drop of sesame oil on the inside of each nostril (and repeat as necessary throughout the day, using almond oil instead if you have sensitive skin).

■ During the flight, stay quiet and avoid conversation. Meditate during take-off and landing. Avoid alcohol, coffee, fizzy drinks, cold food and drinks or wind-producing foods (cabbage, beans, lentils, etc.) and choose warm, easily digested foods instead. Listen to calm, soothing music with your eyes closed and don't be tempted to work during your journey as this will lead to a vata or pitta imbalance and leave you feeling tired and agitated.

■ On the evening of your arrival, have a short walk—preferably in natural surroundings—then fill your bedroom with lavender aroma oil, give yourself an oil massage (paying particular attention to your ears), do your yoga, breathing and meditation routine, have your bedtime drink (see page 62) and go to bed early.

drivers when you take time to check at crossroads and junctions, but you are the least likely dosha to have an accident. You prefer comfort and safety to performance every time, so you will naturally prefer a large car with well-upholstered seats and lots of extra safety features. You are indubitably the best professional driver and you find driving an enjoyable and stimulating experience. Music and energizing oils will make your car journeys even better.

Pittas' competitive nature can make driving a fast and aggressive business—road rage is pure pitta imbalance. You like expensive, top-of-the-range cars for both their speed and their status. While you can become a very skilled driver, you are also the most likely to have a serious accident because of your speed and impatience. You are also the worst passenger—the ultimate back-seat driver who always knows best and is highly critical of others' driving skills. You are an

excellent map-reader, as you take pleasure in detail and precision. Whether you are travelling as driver or passenger, you will benefit from keeping the car cool with the windows open or, in cold weather, from using cooling aroma oils, such as sandalwood or lavender. Play soft, calming music—never fast rock which will overstimulate pitta. Always leave plenty of time for a journey as running late inflames pitta and makes you drive even more recklessly.

Vatas find driving exhausting. Add to this a lack of concentration, a hopeless sense of direction, indecisiveness and a poor sense of spatial awareness and you have the recipe for minor disasters. Vatas tend not to have serious accidents, but you do have lots of lesser scrapes when parking or even getting out of the car—for instance, opening the door without looking. The best way for you to drive is in silence or with soothing, relaxing music, and a vata-pacifying oil in the car. Even better, drive as little as possible, and never talk while you drive.

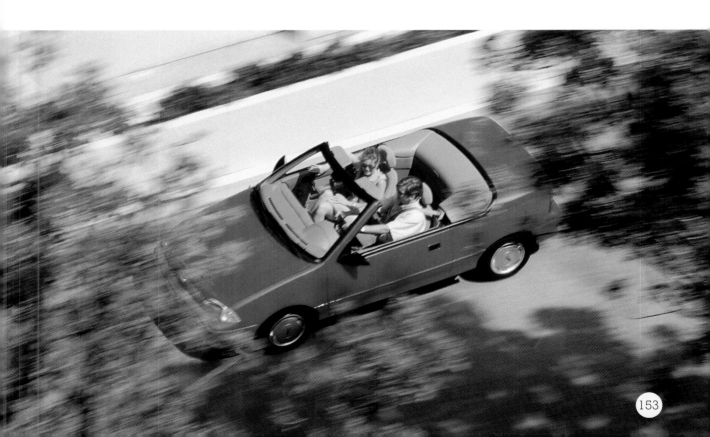

Perfect days

According to European ayurveda, the emotions are an essential factor for well-being. Most people think about this from a negative point of view but, just as negative emotions can be a trigger to disease, so positive ones can affect your health beneficially. Feeling happy, contented and at one with the world should be recognized as a valid aim in itself and, with this in mind, we have created a blueprint for three perfect days, one for each dosha.

Vata's perfect day

■ As you tend to be constantly busy and on the go, your perfect day should be the opposite—a time to relax, chill out and be at peace. You could spend the day completely on your own or, if you prefer, some of the time with a few others in a quiet, focussed activity. However, keep away from crowds and busy places and, if you have to go somewhere by car, ask someone else to drive you.

■ Follow your basic Daily Routine (see pages 108–11) but extend the morning activities to treat yourself to a massage or go to a yoga or meditation class. A day at a spa is often Vata's perfect day, provided that the accent is on peaceful pampering rather than a constant buzz of exertion and activity. Alternatively, if the weather is warm, go for a walk in the countryside or by the sea—somewhere quiet and beautiful. Have your favorite lunch with a partner or a small circle of friends, but avoid noisy restaurants.

■ Vatas are highly artistic and creative activities make you feel calm and confident. You could spend the afternoon painting or drawing, reading or writing, or going to see an inspirational film—nothing violent or scary though!

■ The perfect Vata evening is quiet, calm and relaxed. Sitting in a garden on a warm summer's night, chatting with a friend over a glass of red wine (very settling for Vatas) is ideal. Before you go to bed (go quite early for a good night's sleep), do a slow, easy set of yoga postures and fill your bedroom with lavender aroma oil.

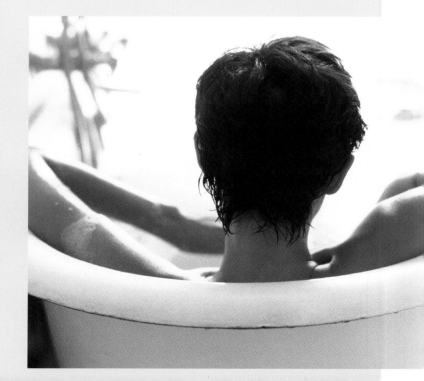

Pitta's perfect day

■ Pitta's perfect day is a busy one with lots of physical and social activity. Follow your basic Daily Routine (see pages 112–5) but make this a fresh-air day as much as possible. If it's hot, don't sit in the sun, but go for cooling environments that still give you the opportunity for plenty of action. Spending a morning swimming, sailing or doing any water sport is ideal, as are skiing, paragliding or hang-gliding (snow and air are both cooling for Pittas). You like a challenge—even an edge of danger —and these sports fulfill that need. If you feel less energetic, though, go for golf, archery, clay-pigeon shooting or a good walk in natural surroundings, ideally by water. Whatever you choose, remember the goal is to have fun—leave your competitive edge at home and just enjoy yourself!

■ Have lunch with a group of friends, if you can in the open air. Don't, however, sit in the sun—find a shady, leafy spot if possible—and avoid alcohol and acidic foods. Have coconut milk and fruit juice instead. Choose sweet, cooling foods and lots of them. Humor is a great tonic for Pittas, so spend the afternoon doing something that makes you laugh. Go to a funny film or a comedy show or read a humorous book. Art galleries, particularly ones featuring paintings or photographs with scenes of natural beauty, are another good option. Finally, you could simply go shopping. Pittas love to shop— good-quality clothes appeal to Pittas' material side and looking good means a lot to you.

■ The evening is definitely party time for Pittas. Social gatherings of any kind, with lively people and stimulating conversation, are ideal for you, but try to relax and don't get too intense. At the very end of the evening, go for a gentle walk—even better when shared with a friend or loved one—to calm you down before sleep.

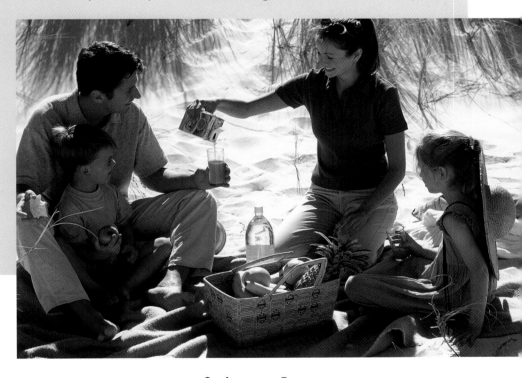

Have lunch with a group of **friends**, if you can in the **open air**.

Kapha's perfect day

■ Start the day early and with a burst of energy—just, in fact, as you mean to go on. Follow your Daily Routine (see pages 116–7) but add in some extra physical activity. Spend an hour in the gym or at an aerobics class, do a weight-training session, or go for a long, vigorous walk or a bike ride. Make sure you do something that stimulates and tests your stamina—really push your boundaries. A demanding team sport, such as rowing or rugby, would make a good alternative. After your exercise session, spend twenty minutes in the steam room.

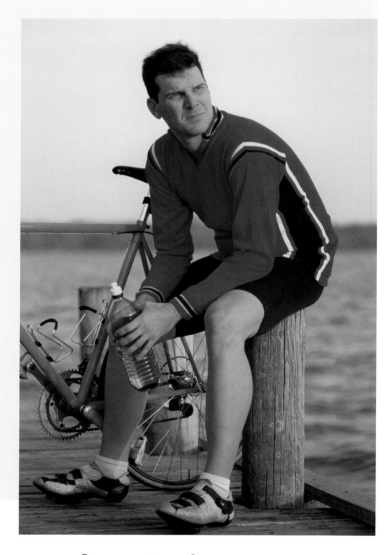

■ Have lunch with friends and choose something hot and spicy like Indian or Mexican, then follow it with a gentle ten- to fifteen-minute walk. In the morning, you stimulated the body and the afternoon is time to stimulate the mind. Spend it playing chess, reading a thriller, playing a quiz game or watching an all-action film. Alternatively, spend the afternoon clearing the decks—throw out anything you no longer use from the attic, the garage or the kitchen drawer. You are a natural hoarder but if you throw away those things you no longer need, you will be amazed at how much fresher you feel mentally.

■ Have a lively evening with family and loved ones. Go dancing, speedway racing or singing with a group of friends. Take a long but gentle walk before retiring for an early night.

Start the day early with a burst of energy —just, in fact, as you mean to go on.

Resources

American Institute of Vedic Studies
PO Box 8357
Santa Fe, NM 87504-8357

AV Products
Dabour India Ltd
101–103 Scrubs Lane
London
NW10 6QU
Tel 0208 960 3960

The Chopra Center for Well Being
7630 Fay Avenue
La Jolla, CA 92037
Tel (619) 551 7788

European Ayurveda Ltd
11 Daryngton Avenue
Birchington
Kent
CT7 9PS
Tel 01843 841010

Index

AUTHOR ACKNOWLEDGMENTS

We would like to thank Colin Beckley, chairman of European Ayurveda Ltd and long-term teacher of transcendental meditation, for his invaluable help on the chapter on meditation. We would also like to thank Carol Willis and Danny Cavanagh for their help with the photograhy and their support throughout, and Colin Larcombe.

I would like to give the biggest thank you to my wife, Terri, for her constant love and support.
(Ian Hayward)

PICTURE CREDITS